TESTIMONIALS

RE: Dr. Rao Konduru's Publications
   1. Permanent Diabetes Control
   2. The Secret to Controlling Type 2 Diabetes
   3. Reversing Obesity
   4. Reversing Sleep Apnea
   5. Reversing Insomnia
   6. Drinking Water Guide

www.drinkingwaterguide.com

TO WHOM IT MAY CONCERN

   Dr. Rao Konduru, PhD is a patient of mine who has suffered from chronic diabetes for most of his life; He also suffered from uncontrollable obesity, sleep apnea and chronic insomnia for the past 3 to 4 years. He has managed to reverse all of these conditions by taking non-pharmacological and science-based natural measures with great success. He has created 6 how-to user guides/books with regard to how he achieved this, and I recommend these books for anyone suffering from these conditions.

Sincerely,
Dr. Ali Ghahary, MD
Brentwood Medical Clinic
4567 Lougheed Hwy
Burnaby, British Columbia, Canada

RE: Permanent Diabetes Control (book)   www.mydiabetescontrol.com

Dr. Konduru is an intelligent and committed scientist who has learned to manage his diabetes and cardiovascular risk factors. This book represents a comprehensive and readable review that could help many people with diabetes.

 Dr. Marshall Dahl
 BSc, MD, PhD, FRCPC, Certified Endocrinologist
 Faculty of Medicine
 University of British Columbia
 Vancouver, British Columbia, Canada

RE: Reversing Sleep Apnea (book)   www.reversingsleepapnea.com

Dear Rao,
I read your book this weekend and it is an impressively comprehensive and extremely well-documented review of the broad spectrum of therapies available to treat and help relieve sleep apnea. You are to be heartily congratulated on a finely-researched and very practical work that will be accessible and useful to a wide audience of readers.
I wish you every success.

Best regards,
 Mr. Martin R. Hoke
 President (Creator and Owner of Navage.com)
 RhinoSystems, Inc.
 Brooklyn Heights, OH-44131
 USA

DRINKING WATER GUIDE

The Quick-Reference Manual to Choosing Clean & Healthy Water

DRINKING WATER GUIDE'S MESSAGE:

- Please do not drink tap water, well water, or bottled water. Please always drink distilled water as is the purest water.

- But distilled water quickly absorbs CO2 from air and forms carbonic acid, making it acidic. So learn how to neutralize it or slightly alkalize it before drinking.

- World Health Organization cautioned that drinking distilled water without minerals in it is harmful to our health (minerals & electrolytes could leach out from body's reservres) so learn how to remineralize it.

- Distilled water that is either neutralized (pH=7) or slightly alkalized (pH=7 to 7.25), and remineralized up to a TDS level of 200 ppm is the healthy drinking water.

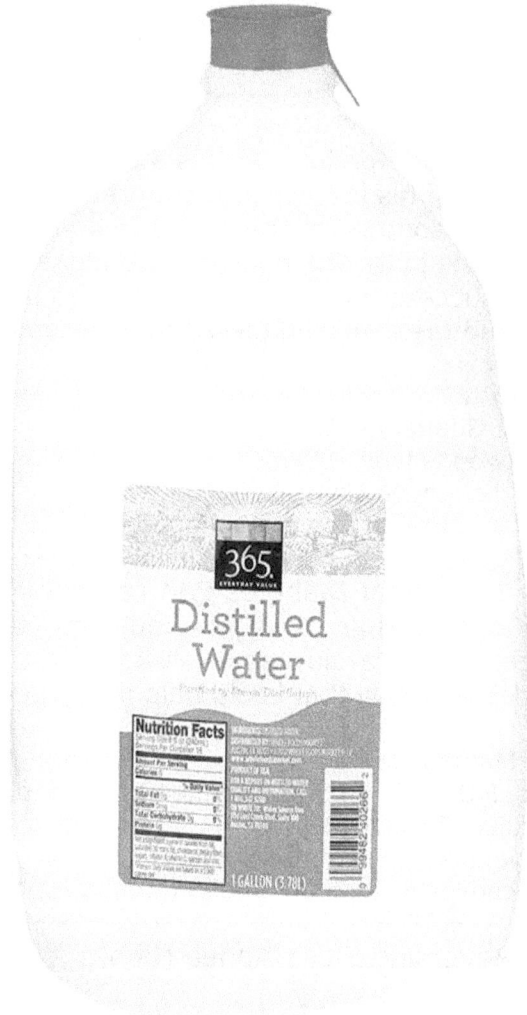

365 EVERYDAY VALUE

Distilled Water

Purified by Steam Distillation

Nutrition Facts

1 GALLON (3.78L)

www.DrinkingWaterGuide.com

Please refer to Chapter 14, Chapter 17, Chapter 18 & Chapter 19 of the complete book "Drinking Water Guide" to learn "how to remineralize and alkalize the purified water at home." There are many experiments conducted at home.

THE ORIGIN OF THE EARTH'S WATER
Formation of Our Universe, Stars, Milky Way Galaxy, Solar System, Sun, Earth & Moon!

This book "The Origin of the Earth's Water" is created with 6 important chapters "Chapter 1, Chapter 2, Chapter 3, Chapter 4, Chapter 14 & Chapter 20" of the complete book "Drinking Water Guide," which has 20 chapters and 540 pages.

This book teaches in Chapter 1 and Chapter 20 "The Formation of Our Universe, Stars, Our Milky Way Galaxy, Our Solar System, Our Sun, Our Earth & Our Moon!"
It also teaches simultaneously the Origin of the Earth's Water. More than 6 billion years ago, even before our Solar System and our Earth were created, hydrogen and oxygen commingled together under the appropriate climate conditions and formed ice-cold water molecules by the chemical reaction $2 H_2 + O_2 = 2 H_2O$, and entered into the space dust and interstellar gas in the interstellar medium, from a gigantic cloud of which our Solar System was created 6 billion years ago. The formation of our Solar System and our Earth completed 4.54 billion years ago.

To Learn "How to Remineralize and Alkalize the Purified Water At Home," please read Page 132, Page 143 and Page 144. Purchase a ZeroWater Pitcher, and make your own purified water from tap water at home. And remieralize and alkalize that purified water before drinking.

DRINKING WATER GUIDE
The Quick-Reference Manual to Choosing Clean & Healthy Water

✓	CHAPTER 1	THE ORIGIN OF THE EARTH'S WATER
✓	CHAPTER 2	DRINKING WATER FACTS & STATISTICS
✓	CHAPTER 3	IMPORTANCE OF DRINKING WATER
✓	CHAPTER 4	TYPES OF DRINKING WATER
	CHAPTER 5	TAP WATER
	CHAPTER 6	BOILED WATER
	CHAPTER 7	BOTTLED WATER
	CHAPTER 8	SPRING WATER
	CHAPTER 9	WELL WATER
	CHAPTER 10	DEMINERALIZED WATER OR DEIONIZED WATER
	CHAPTER 11	REVERSE OSMOSIS WATER
	CHAPTER 12	DESALINATED WATER
	CHAPTER 13	DISTILLED WATER
✓	CHAPTER 14	ZERO WATER, BRITA AND PUR FILTRATION SYSTEMS
	CHAPTER 15	ATMOSPHERIC WATER GENERATORS
	CHAPTER 16	HOW TO SANITIZE REUSABLE WATER BOTTLES
	CHAPTER 17	REMINERALIZATION OF THE PURIFIED WATER
	CHAPTER 18	ALKALINE WATER
	CHAPTER 19	DRINKING WATER GUIDE IN A NUTSHELL
✓	CHAPTER 20	THE ORIGIN OF THE EARTH'S WATER (Continued)

ATTENTION READERS: There Are 3 Books

1. Drinking Water Guide is the 540-page thick book loaded with all 20 chapters. This book describes about all kinds of drinking water available for human consumption (Tap Water, Boiled Water, Bottled Water, Spring Water, Well Water, Demineralized Water, Reverse Osmosis Water, Desalinated Water, Distilled Water, Water from ZeroWater, Brita or PUR pitchers & Water from Atmospheric Water Generators), their defects, and appropriate "RECOMMENDATIONS" on how to rectify those defects, and how to drink clean and healthy water in order to protect your health. In the 2nd part of the book, in Chapter 17, Chapter 18 & Chapter 19, this book teaches "How to Remineralize and Alkalize the Purified Water at Home Correctly and Precisely." There are more than 10 Scientific Experiments Conducted at Home. If you know how to use the TDS meter, digital kitchen scale & digital pH meter, you can easily remineralize and alkalize the purified water at home.

2. Drinking Water Guide-II is the 256-page compacted version, compiled with 8 important chapters (Chapter 1, Chapter 2, Chapter 3, Chapter 4, Chapter 14, Chapter 17, Chapter 18 & Chapter 19). This book is created for those people who cannot afford to purchase the complete book Drinking Water Guide (Paperback). In Chapter 1, this book teaches "The Formation of Our Universe, Stars, Our Milky Way Galaxy, Our Solar System, Our Sun, Our Earth & Our Moon!" based on scientific research findings. In Chapter 2, Chapter 3, Chapter 4, Chapter 14, you will learn about the importance of drinking water, types of drinking water, and how to drink purified water that is properly remineralized and slightly alkalized. If genuine RO water and distilled water are not available in the market, this book suggests that a consumer must switch to zero water. Make your own purified water using a ZeroWater pitcher. And learn how to alkalize and remineralize the zero water at home. Everything is explained clearly in Chapter 14. Just by reading the instructions provided in 2 pages only, you will be able to remineralize and alkalize the purified water (RO water, distilled water, or zero water) like a layperson. In Chapter 17 & Chapter 18, there are more than 10 Scientific Experiments Conducted at Home. Any reasonable person with minimal scientific background will be able to read and understand these experiments.

3. The Origin of the Earth's Water is the 166-page compacted version, compiled with 6 important chapters (Chapter 1, Chapter 2, Chapter 3, Chapter 4, Chapter 14 & Chapter 20). This book is created for those people who are interested on reading the scientific findings about how the planet Earth possessed that much liquid water. In Chapter 1 and Chapter 20, this book teaches "The Formation of Our Universe, Stars, Our Milky Way Galaxy, Our Solar System, Our Sun, Our Earth & Our Moon!" based on scientific research findings. In Chapter 2, Chapter 3, Chapter 4, Chapter 14, you will learn about the importance of drinking water, types of drinking water, and how to drink purified water that is properly remineralized and slightly alkalized. If genuine RO water and distilled water are not available in the market, this book suggests that a consumer must switch to zero water, and must learn how to alkalize and remineralize the zero water at home. Everything is explained clearly in Chapter 14. Just by reading the instructions provided in 2 pages only, you will be able to remineralize and alkalize the purified water (RO water, distilled water, or zero water) like a layperson.

The Big Bang Theory explained in Chapter 1 of the above-mentioned 3 books is the most relevant, most essential, and most important part. In order to understand "The Origin of the Earth's Water," a reader must understand the formation of our Universe, the formation of Stars and the formation of our Solar System, as explained in Chapter 1. This book also teaches in Chapter 1 that all those heavier elements of our periodic table, including all those minerals that we use today to remineralize and alkalize the purified water, were originally manufactured in the burning cores of collapsing stars by a process known as "stellar nucleosynthesis," even before our Solar System and our planet Earth were created. It is therefore of utmost importance to understand, as explained in Chapter 1, the formation of our Universe, the formation of Stars, and the formation our Solar System. All 3 books unveiled, based on scientific findings, the origin of our Earth's water, the age of our Earth's water, the age of our planet Earth, the age of our Sun, the age of our Solar System, and the age of our Milky Way, and the age of our Universe.

DRINKING WATER GUIDE
The Quick-Reference Manual to Choosing Clean & Healthy Water

DRINKING WATER GUIDE'S MESSAGE:

- Please do not drink tap water, well water, or bottled water of any kind directly without knowing how pure it is.

- Please always drink purified water (RO water, distilled water, or zero water), and learn how to remineralize and alkalize the purified water at home.

- Purified water that is either neutralized (pH=7) or slightly alkalized (pH=7 to 7.25), and remineralized up to a TDS (Total Dissolved Solids) level of 200 ppm is the healthy drinking water.

- MAKE YOUR OWN MINERAL WATER: This book teaches everything you need on "how to drink purified water that is remineralized up to 88 trace minerals in it, and slightly alkalized."

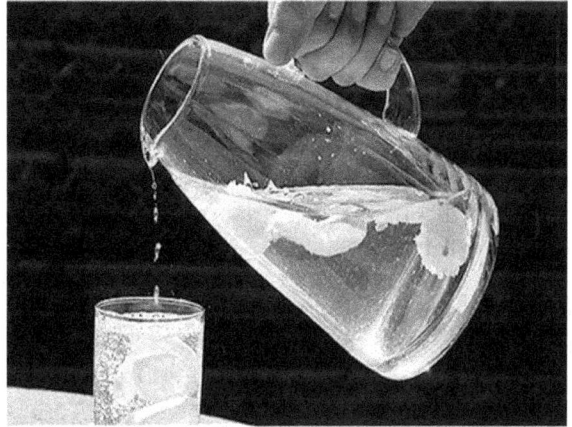

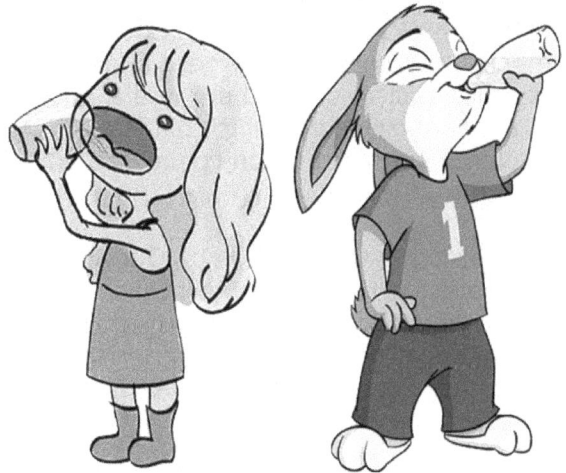

www.DrinkingWaterGuide.com

○ Please refer to Chapter 14, Chapter 17, Chapter 18 & Chapter 19 of the complete book "Drinking Water Guide" to learn "how to remineralize and alkalize the purified water at home." There are many experiments conducted at home.

AMAZON REVIEWS: Drinking Water Guide, Drinking Water Guide-II & The Origin of the Earth's Water

Formation of Our Universe, Stars, Milky Way Galaxy, Solar System, Sun, Earth & Moon!

Please do not ignore reviews. Please read all reviews thoroughly.
You can learn a lot by reading through the reviews below:

Steve_M
5.0 out of 5 stars The Origin of Our Drinking Water Unveiled!
Reviewed in the United States on October 27, 2020
Verified Purchase

Both books Drinking Water Guide and Drinking Water Guide-II clarify that the water formation of our planet Earth occurred in the interstellar medium about 6 billion years ago even before the Solar System formation, and even before the Earth was born. The two essential elements "hydrogen and oxygen" must be available abundantly under appropriate climate conditions to create water molecules. These conditions should suit and encourage the following chemical reaction (two hydrogen molecules combine with one oxygen molecule) to take place naturally in the interstellar medium: $2 H2 + O2 = 2 H2O$

Some 6 billion years ago, when our Solar System was about to form, suitable climate conditions prevailed for the formation of water molecules from the abundantly available elements "hydrogen and oxygen" and entered into the particles of space dust and interstellar gas (also called primordial gas), and remained hidden, in the interstellar medium from a gigantic cloud of which our Solar System was created. About 4.54 billion years ago, our Solar System formation completed, and that is how our Earth possessed liquid water even before it was born.

Very Interesting Observation by Our Astronomers and Space Scientists: NASA reported that there is plenty of water everywhere in the interstellar medium of our Milky Way Galaxy. Which obviously means that there could be liquid water and therefore "the life" similar to our planet Earth on the planets orbiting around the other Solar Systems of our Milky Way Galaxy (there are 500 billion Solar Systems), and even on countless planets of other galaxies across our Universe.

I was blown away by this amazing information revealed in this wonderfully written book of scientific facts and anecdotes regarding the history of water formation on our planet Earth. This book is well-organized by pulling together a compelling story. I commend the author whoever wrote this book!

KON
5.0 out of 5 stars   I enjoyed this book very much!
Reviewed in the United States on December 13, 2019
Format: Kindle Edition
This book is extremely extraordinary, in the wake of perusing this book I am so intrigued. On account of the writer, I would prescribe this book to anybody. Many thanks to the author for giving us such a beautiful book.

Sammantha
5.0 out of 5 stars Awesome Book
Reviewed in the United States on February 18, 2020
Verified Purchase

I appreciated Chapter 1 so much in which the creation and formation of our Universe is described with beautiful depictions and images.

I did not know until I read this book that the water we drink today is 4.54 billion years old. Research proved that our Earth inherited 50% of its water from the interstellar medium, and the remaining water came to Earth from the bombardment of Asteroids (not Comets).

Very interesting to learn that our planet Earth was manufactured by our Sun in a swirling and spinning motion for one and half billion years before the Solar System was ready.

Anamaría Aguirre Chourio
5.0 out of 5 stars Inspiring & Informative Book
Reviewed in the United States on February 19, 2020
Verified Purchase

The first chapter is inspiring and lovely. Our Universe, our Stars, our Milky Way Galaxy, our Solar System, our Sun, our Planet Earth & our Moon: How were they created? This book answered that question clearly with amazing descriptions based on scientific research.

Common sense tells that Earth could have gotten water from an external source such as comets, asteroids or meteorites such as carbonecious chondrites, which contain water as well as carbon. It was known to scientists that our planet Earth was bombarded by comets, asteroids and meteorites (such as carbonecious chondrites). If water came from the dirty ice-balls, then comets are logical candidates for the existence of water on Earth, but scientists proved that the Deuterium-to-Hydrogen Ratio (D/H Ratio) on comets is too high, and did not match with that of sea water.

The researchers were able to match the Deuterium-to-Hydrogen Ratio (D/H Ratio) between the sea water and the water samples from Asteroids (specifically carbonecious chondrites). Which means that the Earth could have accreted at least 50% of its water from Asteroids during the early states after its formation. Our Earth already inherited up to 50% of its water from interstellar medium even before it was created in our Solar System. I am glad that I learned the aforementioned very important scientific truth from this book.

Deanna Maio
5.0 out of 5 stars <u>Wonderful Book</u>
Reviewed in the United States on February 17, 2020
Verified Purchase

Comets did not contribute to the water formation on the Earth. This book explores that Asteroids contributed to the water formation on the Earth about 4.54 billion years ago (which is the age of our Solar System, Our Sun & Our Earth). Based on scientific research findings, this book explores that our Earth inherited up to 50% of its water from the interstellar medium even before its birth.

Our Solar System was created from a gigantic cloud of space dust & gas of a deceased star some 6 billion years ago in the interstellar medium. At that time that space dust and gas of the interstellar medium already filled with water, and enter into the planet Earth during its formation. It is a fascinating book, and I feel like reading it over and over again.

Jack mckeever
5.0 out of 5 stars Amazing Scientific Book, Strongly Recommended!
Reviewed in the United Kingdom on 1 May 2020
Verified Purchase

I learned a very important information from this book. Water forms anywhere in our Milky Way Galaxy and in our Universe as long as the appropriate conditions prevail:

(i) Both hydrogen and oxygen must abundantly be available under appropriate climate conditions (temperatures below 50 °K may be necessary in most cases), and
(ii) The ionization of hydrogen molecules should readily be possible in order to take place the chemical reaction ($2 H_2 + O_2 = 2 H_2O$).

Nearly 380,000 years after the Big Bang, hydrogen was the most common and dominant element, abundantly available in our Universe. Nearly 400 million years after the Big Bang, stars formation commenced. The massive pressure build-up of the fiery inferno within the stars is so great that hydrogen atoms fused together to form heavier element helium, and helium atoms in turn fused together to form much heavier elements like lithium, beryllium, carbon, nitrogen and oxygen in a process called "nucleosynthesis". The early stars were massive and short-lived. When the massive stars finished burning their hydrogen or helium fuel, eventually extinguished, collapsed and exploded into supernovae. These new elements "helium, carbon, nitrogen, oxygen, and other elements" along with hydrogen from Big Bang were spread across the galaxies throughout our Universe. During the supernova explosions, these elements combined together to form all kinds of new elements that we see in the periodic table today.

At that time, when new elements were being formed, hydrogen and oxygen could have combined together and formed water molecules by the chemical reaction ($2 H_2 + O_2 = 2 H_2O$), and could have entered the gigantic cloud of space dust and primordial gas from which our solar system (our Sun, our planet Earth & other 7 planets) was created.

A Collins
5.0 out of 5 stars Very Important Book
Reviewed in Canada on February 15, 2020
Verified Purchase

This book describes the creation and formation of our Universe and our Solar System impressively with amazing descriptions based on scientific research. This book presents scientific data collected by NASA's scientists and space researchers regarding the origin of the Earth's water. The majority of scientific studies convincingly revealed the fact that our planet Earth inherited up to 50% of its water from the interstellar medium even before its birth, and the remaining water was believed and proved to have obtained from the bombardment of asteroids (meteorites/ carbonaceous chondrites) during the early stages of the formation of our planet Earth in the solar system. The scientific data on deuterium-hydrogen ratio (D/H Ratio) collected by our researchers supported this conclusion.

The water we drink today is 4.54 billion years old, which is also the age of our planet EARTH. I love this book!

---

stacy anderson
5.0 out of 5 stars The Origin of the Earth's Water Is Revealed in This Book!
Reviewed in the United Kingdom on June 9, 2021
Verified Purchase

This book revealed the scientific truth in detail in Chapter 1 & Chapter 20. The water we drink today is at least 4.54 billion years old, older than our planet Earth, older than our Sun, and older than our Solar System. Our planet Earth inherited roughly 50% of its water from the interstellar medium even before it was born, and the rest of the water came to our planet Earth by the bombardment of Asteroids. Those Asteroids of course inherited their water even before our Solar System was created. Our ancestors' belief that Comets brought water to our planet Earth was later proved by our scientists to be a myth.

Our Solar System was created from a gigantic cloud of space dust and the interstellar gas in the interstellar medium, which already contained water molecules in it. The author dedicated Chapter 1 & Chapter 20 to explain everything about it with scientific details, including the formation of our Universe, the formation of Stars, the formation of our Milky Way Galaxy, the formation of our Solar System, and the formation Water even before our Solar System was created.

This book cautions everybody: "Please do not drink tap water, well water, or bottled water of any kind without knowing how pure it is."

This book recommends everybody: "Please always drink purified water (RO water or distilled water)." And learn how to remineralize and alkalize the purified water at home.

HOW TO REMINERALIZE & ALKALIZE THE PURIFIED WATER AT HOME! PLEASE READ CHAPTER 14

Peggie Tyson
5.0 out of 5 stars Why remineralize and alkalize the purified water at home?
Reviewed in the United States on June 29, 2022
Verified Purchase

Why remineralize and alkalize the purified water at home?

This book answered that question very clearly. World Health Organization (WHO) cautioned repeatedly long ago that drinking demineralized water (RO water, distilled water, zero water, or any other purified water) is harmful to our health because certain scientific investigations revealed the fact that minerals and electrolytes could leach out from body's reserves and cause strange diseases and many abnormalities if there are not enough minerals and electrolytes present in the drinking water. We therefore must learn how to precisely remineralize the purified water before drinking.

Also purified water quickly absorbs carbon dioxide (CO_2) from the surrounding air and forms carbonic acid, making it acidic. The pH of purified water may drop to as low as 5.6, making it dangerously acidic. We therefore must also learn how to neutralize (pH=7) or slightly alkalize (pH=7 to 7.25) the purified water before drinking.

HIMALAYAN PINK SALT, CELTIC SEA SALT, CONCENTRACE MINERAL DROPS & BAKING SODA: Himalayan pink salt contains 88 trace minerals in it, and attributes to many health benefits. Himalayan pink salt also contains six electrolytes "sodium, potassium, chloride, magnesium, phosphorus and calcium" in it. Our bodies desperately need all these 6 electrolytes. Celtic sea salt contains 72 trace mineral in it, and ConcenTrace mineral drops contains 73 trace minerals in it. All these products are claimed to have the essential electrolytes in them. Baking soda is the best alkalizing agent.

We can very easily remineralize the purified water to any desired TDS level by adding the precisely measured tiny amount of Himalayan pink salt, Celtic sea salt, ConcenTrace mineral drops. ConcenTrace mineral drops can be used to simultaneously remineralize and alkalize the purified water (RO water, Distilled Water, or Zero Water) at home. We can very easily alkalize the purified water by adding a trace amount (only a few kernels) of baking soda.

This awesome book presented many experiments conducted at home on how to remineralize and alkalize the purified water at home using TDS meter, digital kitchen scale and digital pH meter. And I am using those experiments.

Anamaría Aguirre Chourio
5.0 out of 5 stars Best Drinking Water Guide to Live Healthy!
Reviewed in the United States on March 18, 2020
Verified Purchase

Drinking Water Guide-II would certainly benefit many people in the way we never have imagined. Everyone should listen to the most important message of this book "Please do not drink tap water, well water & bottled water. Please always drink purified water, and learn how to remineralize and alkalize the purified water at home." This book has guided me and taught me many healthy water-drinking habits, and I list some of them below:

(i) I purchased a Countertop Water Distiller (the same distiller recommended in this book), and I now make my own distilled water every day. No more tap water.

(ii) I also purchased ConcenTrace mineral drops from a health food store near me.

(iii) I also purchased a TDS meter (the same meter recommended in this book) from Amazon. I learned how to use it from this book.

(iv)) I also purchased a Digital pH Meter (the same meter recommended in this book) from Amazon. I learned how to use it from this book.

(v) I have read Chapter 17, Chapter 18 & Chapter 19 several times. It was very easy to read and understand procedures. In Chapter 17, I read that: An adult must drink at least 8 cups or 2 liters of purified water, and so 16 drops of ConcenTrace mineral drops are required per day to remineralize the purified water to keep the TDS level under 200 ppm, and to keep the drinking water slightly alkalized.

(vi) Every day, when I wake up in the morning, I mix 16 drops of ConcenTrace mineral drops with 2 liters (8 cups) of distilled water, and I drink all 8 cups throughout the day. The water I drink thus is purified, remineralized up to 200 ppm, and slightly alkalized as well (this is perfectly healthy water).

The manufacturer of ConcenTrace mineral drops recommends 40 drops per day without specifying the total number of cups of water to be mixed with per day. But this book recommends that more than 16 drops per 2 liters of purified water would be unnecessary, and may develop life-threatening long-term side effects because of high sodium consumption (I fully agree!).

I am sure that these water-drinking habits would keep me in good health. I now know that I would not become a victim of contaminated drinking water (mostly tap water), and will not develop any strange diseases due to mineral deficiency, and my body's cells would not leach minerals like some scientists claim.

Amazon Customer
5.0 out of 5 stars How to Remineralize Purified Water Like a Layperson?
Reviewed in India on October 2, 2022
Verified Purchase

I have read just 2-page instructions titled "How to Alkalize and Remineralize Like a Layperson?" very kindly provided in the beginning of Chapter 17. That information is enough for me to remineralize and alkalize the purified water.

TRIAL AND ERROR PROCEDURE

(i) Every day I make "4 liters (16 cups)" of purified water using a zero water pitcher, and store it in a glass bottle. I add only a few kernels of Himalayan pink salt to this zero water, shake the glass bottle vigorously and monitor the TDS level using the TDS meter that comes "attached" with the zero water pitcher. The TDS level is usually close to 10 ppm.
(ii) I add a few more kernels of Himalayan pink salt, shake the glass bottle vigorously and monitor TDS level again. The TDS level is usually close to 20 ppm.
(iii) I add a few more kernels of Himalayan pink salt, shake the glass bottle vigorously and monitor TDS level again. The TDS level is usually close to 30 ppm. This is my desired TDS level.
(iv) I boil this remineralized zero water using a glass kettle, and refrigerate it before drinking.
(v) Every day I drink 10 to 16 cups of purified water (zero water) remineralized to a TDS level of approximately 30 ppm. Drinking lots of pure water helps me lose weight, and keeps my weight normal.
(vi) I do not try to alkalize the purified water (zero water), but I eat 1 lemon a day. That keeps my body at neutralized state (my urine pH close to 7). I will continue drinking this kind of purified and remineralized water for the rest of my life. I am sure this habit will keep my body healthy.

I am greatly indebted to this extremely important book "Drinking Water Guide-II: How to Remineralize and Alkalize the Purified Water At Home."

Harish Garg
5.0 out of 5 stars Extremely Important Guide to Remineralize and Alkalize the Purified Water!
Reviewed in India on July 27, 2022
Verified Purchase

Drinking Water Guide-II contains extremely important and beneficial information to remineralize and alkalize the purified water at home. I found it extremely useful and helpful.

(i) With the help of this book, I purchased a ZeroWater pitcher and started making my own zero water from tap water. Zero water is better than distilled water because the distilled water being sold in supermarkets is untrustworthy (as it could have scum in it). Zero water has a TDS level of zero so we must remineralize it before drinking according to World Health Organization (WHO).

(ii) With the help of this book, after reading the experiments conducted at home, I added a tiny pinch (only a few kernels) of Himalayan pink salt to zero water so that TDS level is approximately 20 ppm. I monitored TDS level of zero water using the TDS meter that comes with the ZeroWater pitcher.

(iii) With the help of this book, after reading the experiments conducted at home, I added a tiny pinch (only a few kernels) of baking soda so that the pH of the zero water would be approximately 7. I measured the pH level of zero water using a digital pH meter as explained in this book. I also learned how to use "pH drops" to measure zero water pH.

(iv) With the help of this book, after reading the experiments conducted at home, I often measure my urine pH using "pH paper for urine," and make sure that it is close to 7. That means my urine is neither acidic nor alkaline, but it is neutralized. Whenever my urine pH is more than 8, I discontinue adding baking soda to the zero water until my urine pH comes down close to 7.

I drink every day at least 8 cups of zero water that is remineralized and either neutralized or slightly alkalized. I learned all the aforementioned drinking water strategies from this great guidebook "Drinking Water Guide-II."

Anoop J.
5.0 out of 5 stars   Remineralization of the Purified Water is Simplified!
Reviewed in India on October 6, 2022
Verified Purchase

REMINERALIZATION OF THE PURIFIED WATER IS SIMPLIFIED:

After I read this book's experiments conducted at home in Chapter 14 & Chapter 17, I developed my own simplified method to remineralize the purified water as explained below.

I purchased a countertop water distiller, and I make my own distilled water enough for a week, every week, and I store it in glass bottles. Did you know the distilled water must be stored in glass bottles with lid?

Every day I pour about 4 liters of distilled water in a glass container with lid, and start adding Himalayan pink salt. I add only a few kernels of Himalayan pink salt, mix and shake the water bottle thoroughly, and monitor the TDS level using the TDS meter. If the TDS level is less than 50 ppm, I add a few more kernels of Himalayan pink salt, mix and shake the water bottle thoroughly, and monitor the TDS level again using the TDS meter. I repeat this procedure until the TDS level of distilled water reaches approximately 50 ppm. I drink at least 8 cups of this remineralized distilled water at 50 ppm.

The most fascinating fact is that I spend less than 2 minutes to remineralize the purified water at my home. Many people think that remineralization is a complex process, and don't even try to do it. The same procedure can be used to remineralize any kind of purified water (RO water, distilled water, or zero water) to any desired TDS level. Everybody in my family circle and many of friends adopted this procedure, and every day, they all make and drink the remineralized distilled water at 50 ppm.

Deanna Maio
5.0 out of 5 stars   Comprehensive Drinking Water Guide
Reviewed in the United States on February 17, 2020
Verified Purchase

NIKOLA TESLA said it all: "only a lunatic will drink unsterilized water". Very many people are still drinking unsterilized tap water and contaminated bottled water, jeopardizing their health, and developing strange diseases, and making many trips to hospitals and board-certified doctors. The tap water disaster incident that occurred in Flint, Michigan, USA in 2014 is a typical example of lead contamination that affected more than 100,000 residents.

This book describes about all kinds of drinking water available for human consumption, their defects, and appropriate "recommendations" in order to rectify those defects, and how to drink clean and healthy water in order to protect your health in the current day circumstances. This book Drinking Water Guide teaches many drinking water strategies:

(i) I must be wise and cautious all the time and should not take chances. I must not drink tap water, well water or bottled water of any kind, and make my own distilled water by purchasing and using a home distiller. Or, I must purchase RO water from a nearby supermarket, and I must always drink only purified water.

(ii) I would add very little Himalayan pink salt, Celtic sea salt or a few drops of ConcenTrace mineral drops to remineralize the purified water before drinking.

(iii) I would add a tiny bit of baking soda or a few drops of ConcenTrace mineral drops in order to improve the alkalinity and the presence of minerals in the purified water.

(iv) I would use pH strips or digital pH meter, monitor my drinking water pH, every now and then, and make sure that the purified water I drink is either neutralized (pH=7) or slightly alkalized (pH=7 to 7.5).

(v) I would use a TSD meter, and monitor the TDS level of my drinking water, and make sure that TDS level is always below 200 ppm. I will also research and find out the ideal TDS level that suits my body. I can do that by adjusting the tiny amount of Himalayan pink salt.

I am very grateful that I learned all the above-mentioned valuable information from this book "Drinking Water Guide". What an impressive book! I urge you to get this book without any hesitation.

DRINKING WATER GUIDE
The Quick-Reference Manual to Choosing Clean & Healthy Water

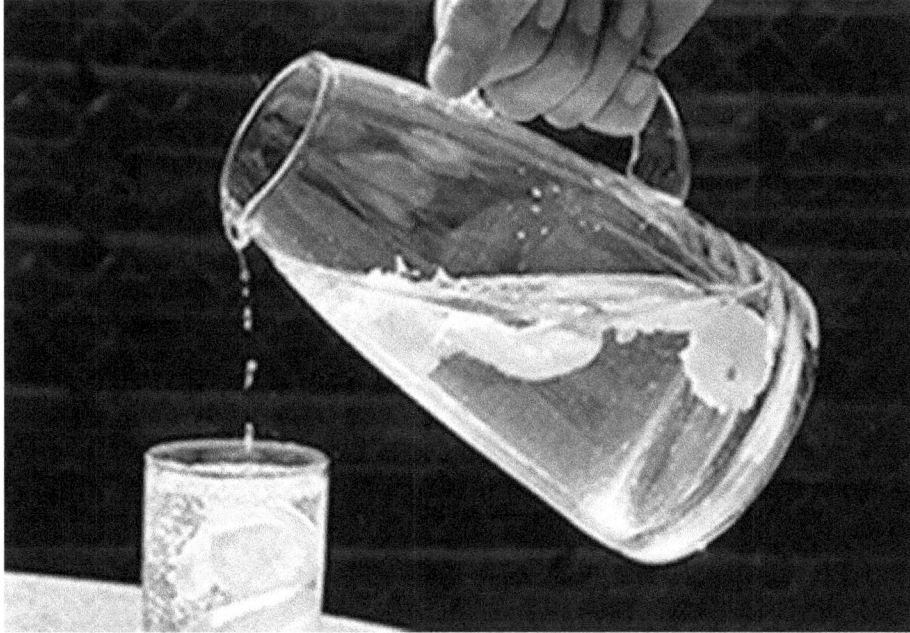

DRINKING WATER GUIDE REMINDS YOU

- Protect Your Health From Strange Water-Borne Diseases!
- Tap Water, Well Water & Bottled Water Are Filled With Contaminants!
- Spring Water Is Collected From Depleted Aquifers & Is Not Purified!
- Please Always Drink Purified Water: RO Water, Or Distilled Water!
- Learn How to Remineralize & Alkalize the Purified Water at Home!

DRINKING WATER GUIDE TEACHES YOU

- Formation Of Our Universe, Our Milky Way Galaxy, Our Sun, Our Earth & Our Moon!
- How In Our Universe Our Earth Possessed That Much Liquid Water?
- How To Remineralize & Alkalize: Experiments Conducted At Home!
- How To Obtain Alkaline Water: There Are 10 Methods Discussed!
- Water Ionizers | Kangen Water | Hydrogen Water | Atmospheric Water
- How To Make Your Own Nutritious Alkaline & Mineral Water At Home!
- How To Adjust the Drinking Water pH and TDS to Any Desired Level!

This Guide Will Help You Become A Drinking Water Expert!
Author: Rao Konduru, PhD

DRINKING WATER GUIDE
The Quick-Reference Manual to Choosing Clean & Healthy Water
Authored by Rao Konduru, PhD

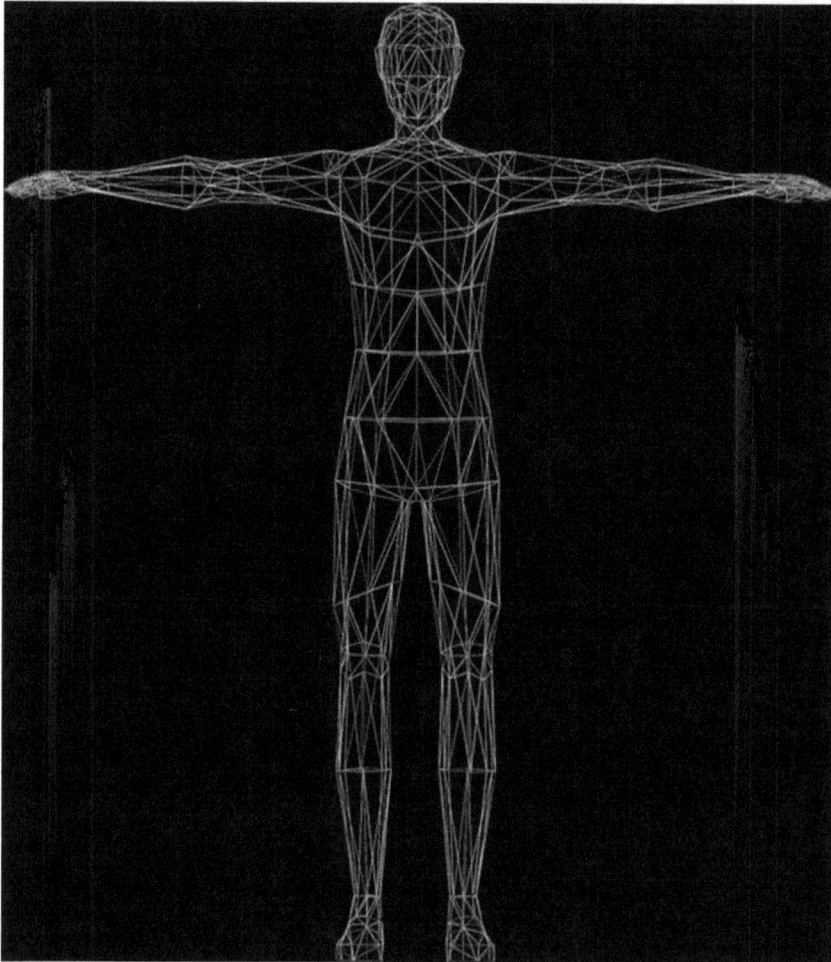

THE AMAZING HUMAN BODY

🌑 Did you know more than 99% of your amazing body's molecules are water molecules, and 55% to 60% of your body weight is water? You therefore should make sure that the water in your body is clean, healthy and nutritious, and more importantly one 100% free of contaminants. This book is designed to help you achieve that goal!

THE ORIGIN OF THE EARTH'S WATER

Formation of Our Universe, Stars, Milky Way Galaxy, Solar System, Sun, Earth & Moon!

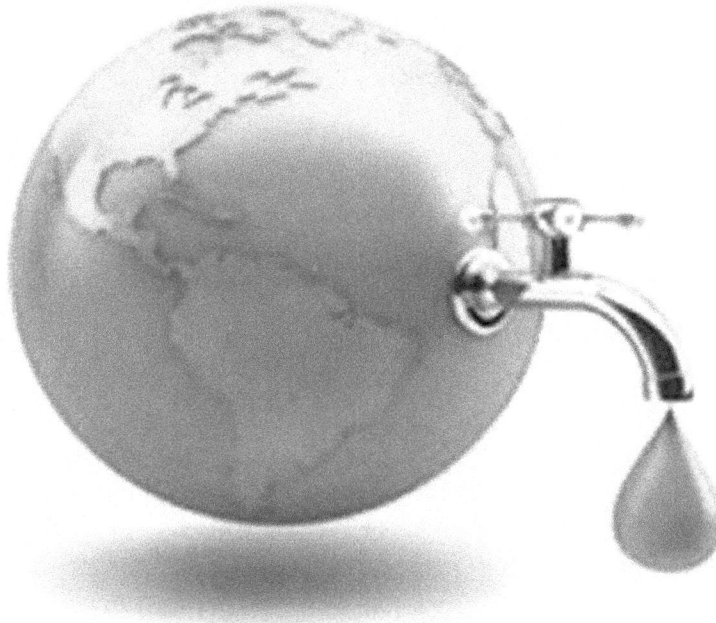

FORMATION OF OUR UNIVERSE

- Formation of Our Universe After The Big Bang 13.8 Billion Years Ago!
- Formation of Our Stars (There Are At Least 10 Billion Trillion Stars)!
- Formation of Our Spiral-Shaped Milky Way Galaxy!
- Did You Know Our Sun Manufactured Our Solar System?
- Formation of Our Solar System: Our Sun, Our Earth & Our Moon!
- Formation of Water On Our Planet Earth!
- Drinking Water Facts, Statistics, Importance and Types!

THEORIES OF WATER FORMATION

- Comets Could Have Brought Water to Our Planet Earth!
- Asteroids Could Have Brought Water to Our Planet Earth!
- Earth Inherited Its Water From The Interstellar Medium!
- Earth's Deep Mantle Has The Water From The Interstellar Medium!
- Earth's Thick Hydrogen Layer Could Have Reacted With Oxygen!
- Which Theory Is Proved To Be True and Which Theory Is False?

Rao Konduru, PhD

"The Origin of the Earth's Water" is only a part (5 Chapters)
of the complete book "Drinking Water Guide," which has 20 Chapters.

PREFACE: "THE ORIGIN OF THE EARTH'S WATER"

THEORIES OF WATER FORMATION ON OUR EARTH	CONCLUSION
1. COMETS COULD HAVE BROUGHT WATER TO EARTH ⚇ Our Solar System (Our Sun, Our Earth and other 7 Planets) began its formation 6 billion years ago, and completed its formation 4.54 billion years ago. Our ancestors believed that ice-bearing comets probably bombarded our Earth 4 to 3.8 billion years ago, and brought water to Earth. This theory is now believed to be wrong because (D/H Ratio) of the water from comets is much higher than that of ocean water. Our ancestors' belief that comets brought water to our planet Earth was however proved by our most recent scientists to be a myth.	MYTH!
2. ASTEROIDS (METEORITES /CARBONACEOUS CHONDRITES) COULD HAVE BROUGHT WATER TO EARTH ⚇ Water-rich asteroids (meteorites / carbonaceous chondrites) impacted the infant Earth about 4 to 3.8 billion years ago, distributing water across the planet by brute force. As a result, our oceans formed. This theory is more accurate because D/H Ratio of the water from asteroids matched well with that of ocean water. Research proved that our planet Earth attained up to 50% of its water from the asteroids during the early stages after the formation of our Solar System.	TRUE!
3. EARTH INHERITED ITS WATER FROM THE INTERSTELLAR MEDIUM ⚇ Water is known to form in the clouds of gas and dust of the interstellar medium (ISM). Our Solar System was created 6 billion years ago from a gigantic cloud of interstellar gas and stardust. That cloud collapsed and formed a solar nebula—a spinning, swirling disk of material under gravity. Scientists found that the primordial water of the interstellar medium survived within the particles of the stardust, and carried forward all the way until and after the formation our Earth. Researchers concluded, from an extensive experimental study and mathematical modelling, that our planet Earth inherited up to 50% of its water from the interstellar medium even before our Solar System was created. Our Solar System completed its formation 4.54 billion years ago. ⚇ However the water we drink today is at least 4.54 billion years old.	TRUE!
4. EARTH'S DEEP MANTLE HAS THE PRIMORDIAL WATER FROM THE INTERSTELLAR MEDIUM ⚇ The researchers collected samples of primitive rocks from the Baffin Island, Nunavut Territory, Canada back in 1985. Water analysis revealed that these rocks have lower amount of deuterium, and lower D/H Ratio, indicating that the Earth's deep mantle attained the primordial water from the interstellar medium. ⚇ Which means the water we drink today is at least 4.54 billion years old.	TRUE!
5. THICK HYDROGEN LAYER COULD HAVE REACTED WITH OXYGEN ⚇ Hydrogen could have reacted with oxygen available from the oxides of Earth's mantle, and could have formed water molecules after our Solar System formed. This water from the mantle could have been later transported to the Earth's surface, forming oceans. [$2 H_2 + O_2 = 2 H_2O$] ⚇ This theory does not have much supporting evidence and so disregarded.	FALSE!

Please refer to Chapter 20 and read through the details of these 5 therories.

ATTENTION READERS!

**Drinking Water Guide Unveiled "The Origin of the Earth's Water"
In Chapter 1 & Chapter 20.**

In CHAPTER 1 & CHAPTER 20,
You Will Learn All About
The Origin of the Earth's Water.

CHAPTER 1 CONTAINS THE PRECIOUS INFORMATION

🌐 Chapter 1 contains the precious information. The Big Bang Theory explained in Chapter 1 of the book is the most relevant, most essential, and most important part. This book teaches that all those heavier elements of our periodic table, including all those minerals that we use today to remineralize and alkalize the purified water, were originally manufactured in the burning cores of collapsing stars by a process known as "stellar nucleosynthesis," even before our Solar System and our planet Earth were created. Stars are responsible for all the constituents of our planet Earth (Carbon, Hydrogen, Nitrogen, Oxygen, Phosphorus and Sulfur are the most important elements) that are needed for the formation and survival of every human being, animal and plant.

In CHAPTER 2, CHAPTER 3, CHAPTER 4 & CHAPTER 14,
You Will Learn Water Statistics, Types of Drinking Water,
Importance of Drinking Water, and
How to Drink Only Purified Water
That is Properly Remineralized and Slightly Alkalized.

In Addition, At The End of This Book,
There Is Bonus Reading from Chapter 17 & Chapter 18.

Remineralization and Alkalization Methods
Are Simplified and Explained Briefly in 2 Pages.

By Reading These 2 Pages Only,
You Can Remineralize and Alkalize The Purified Water
(RO Water, Distilled Water, or Zero Water)
Like a Layperson at Home and Enjoy Mineral Water!

MAKE YOUR OWN NUTRITIOUS MINERAL WATER!
It Is Very Easy to Remineralize and Alkalize!
[You Don't Have to Read all Scientific Experiments!]

Purified water (zero water) that is either neutralized (pH=7) or slightly alkalized (pH= 7 to 7.5), and remineralized up to a TDS level of 200 ppm is the healthy drinking water.

◉ The primary element "hydrogen" was first created 380,000 years after the Big Bang, and thereafter it was abundantly available throughout our Universe. Stars formation commenced 400 million years after the Big Bang, and since then stars have been manufacturing heavier elements, including the very important oxygen, like factories in their burning cores, and have been dumping them in the interstellar medium via supernova explosions. More than 6 billion years ago, even before our Solar System and our Earth were created, the heavier element "oxygen" was created in the burning cores of collapsing stars in the interstellar medium.

◉ The abundantly available hydrogen and oxygen then commingled together under the appropriate climate conditions and formed ice-cold water molecules by the chemical reaction: $2 H_2 + O_2 = 2 H_2O$. Those ice-cold water molecules then entered into the space dust (also known as stardust) and interstellar gas in the interstellar medium, from a gigantic cloud of which our Solar System was created 6 billion years ago. The formation of our Solar System completed 4.54 billion years ago. And that is how our Earth inherited liquid water even before it was born. Our Earth was thus born with water, and the water we drink today is at least 4.54 billion years old, older than our Solar System.

◉ In order to understand "The Origin of the Earth's Water," a reader must understand, as explained in Chapter 1, the formation of our Universe, the formation of Stars, and the formation of our Solar System with a clear concept.

◉ This book also revealed, based on brilliant scientific findings, the age of our Earth's water, the age of our planet Earth, the age of our Sun, the age of our Solar System, the age of our Milky Way Galaxy, and the age of our Universe.

◉ **The Big Bang Theory Explained in Chapter 1** is the most relevant, the most essential, and the most intriguing part of this book. Stars are responsible for all the constituents of our planet Earth that are needed for the formation and survival of every human being, animal and plant. Did you know "the oxygen we breathe today was originally created in the Stars even before our Solar System was created, and the water we drink today was originally created in the stars-forming clouds even before our Solar System was created?" This book teaches that all those heavier elements of our periodic table, including the most important carbon, nitrogen, oxygen, phosphorus, sulfur, and other elements, and including all those minerals that we use today to remineralize and alkalize the purified water, were originally manufactured in the burning cores of collapsing stars by a process known as "stellar nucleosynthesis," even before our Solar System and our Earth were created. When you look up at night, you are seeing factories called stars.

◉ It is therefore of utmost importance to understand, as explained in Chapter 1, the formation of our Universe, the formation of Stars, and the formation our Solar System.

Please read and understand CHAPTER 1 with keen observation, and understand the Big Bang Therory. Please read and understand CHAPTER 20 with keen observation, and understand the theories of water formation on our planet Earth. At the end of CHAPTER 20, please read the CONCLUSIONS regarding the water formation.

-- The Author

COPYRIGHT

PLEASE NOTE: "The Origin of the Earth's Water" is the compacted version of the original book "Drinking Water Guide", which has 20 chapters and 540 pages.
"The Origin of the Earth's Water" is compiled with 6 important chapters of the original book "Drinking Water Guide": Chapter 1, Chapter 2, Chapter 3, Chapter 4, Chapter 14 and Chapter 20.

Book Title: **The Origin of the Earth's Water**
Sub-Title: Formation of Our Universe, Stars, Milky Way Galaxy, Solar System, Sun, Earth & Moon!
Author: Rao Konduru, PhD (Also Called Dr. RK)
Publisher: Prime Publishing Co.
Address: 720 – Sixth Street, Unit: 161
New Westminster, BC, Canada, V3L 3C5
Website: www.drinkingwaterguide.com
ISBN # ISBN 9780973112085

This book "The Origin of the Earth's Water" has been registered under ISBN Number "ISBN 9780973112085" with the National Library of Canada Cataloguing in Publication, Ottawa, Ontario, Canada. The original manuscript has been submitted to the Legal Deposits, Library and Archives Canada, Ottawa, Ontario, Canada. All rights reserved!

WARNING

DISCLAIMER

The author of the books titled "Drinking Water Guide" and "The Origin of the Earth's Water" assumes no liability or responsibility including, without limitation, incidental and consequential damages, personal injury or wrongful death resulting from the use of any treatment method presented in this book. All contents in these books are for educational purpose only, and do not in any way represent the professional medical advice.

REGARDING THE REFERENCES

Please note that the hypelinks of the references provided in all chapters are not guaranteed to work. The owners of those websites might have changed the contents, and some of those websites might have even disappeared from the Internet. However the information collected from all the scientific articles and journal papers was found to be true and reliable at the time the literature search was performed.

TABLE OF CONTENTS

CHAPTER 1 THE ORIGIN OF THE EARTH'S WATER
EARTH GOT ITS WATER EVEN BEFORE IT WAS BORN

TABLE OF CONTENTS

Did you know?
The oxygen we breathe today was originally created in the Stars
even before our Solar System was created!
The water we drink today was originally created in the stars-forming clouds
even before our Solar System was created!
When you look up at night, you are seeing factories called Stars!

AMAZING FACTS ABOUT OUR UNIVERSE, OUR STARS, OUR MILKY WAY GALAXY, OUR SOLAR SYSTEM, OUR SUN, OUR EARTH & OUR WATER!

The following scientific facts were endorsed by NASA (National Aeronautics and Space Administration) and many other space agencies around the world:

- <u>Our Universe is approximately 13.8 billion years old.</u> [1, 2, 3, 4, 5]
  The NASA's spacecraft known as Wilkinson Microwave Anisotropy Probe (WMAP) mission has precisely determined the age of our Universe.

- <u>Our Universe has trillion trillion stars</u>. [6, 7]
  There are 1,000,000,000,000,000,000,000,000 stars. There are 10^{24} stars. [6, 7]
  That's is a 1 followed by twenty-four zeros.
  This is a grossly rough estimate. The exact number of stars is unknown.

- <u>Our Universe is embedded with at least 2 trillion Galaxies.</u> There are 2×10^{12} Galaxies. [8, 9, 10]
  <u>The Spiral-Shaped Milky Way Galaxy is one of them upon which we all live</u>.
- <u>Our Milky Way Galaxy was born about 13.6 billion years ago.</u> [11, 12, 13]
- <u>Our Milky Way Galaxy has 100 billion stars on the lower end, and 400 billion stars on the upper end, totaling at least 500 billion stars</u>. [14]
- Did you know every star represents a Solar System with planets orbiting around it?
- <u>That means our Milky Way Galaxy so far has at least 500 billion Solar Systems.</u> [14, 15, 16]
  <u>Our Solar System is one of them</u>.

- <u>Our Solar System (our Sun, our Earth & 7 other planets)</u> began its formation on our Milky Way Galaxy 6 billion years ago, and completed its formation 4.54 billion years ago. [55-60]
- <u>Did you know stars manufacture planets?</u> Our Sun (which is a star) manufactured 8 orbiting planets "Mercury, Venus, our Earth, Mars, Jupiter, Saturn, Uranus and Neptune" while in a spinning and swirling motion under gravity for one and half billion years. [55-60]

- The age of our planet Earth, our Sun & our Solar System was determined by radiometric dating, which is the most accurate and reliable technique to date older rocks. [65-71]
- <u>Did you know stars manufacture heavier elements like factories do?</u> When you look up at night, you are seeing factories called stars equipped with nuclear-fusion reactors! [39, 40, 41]
- Early stars were massive, short-lived and exploded into supernovae while manufacturing and dumping all those 117 heavier elements of our periodic table into the interstellar space from a gigantic cloud of which our Solar System was created! The SIX essential elements "Carbon, Hydrogen, Nitrogen, Oxygen, Phosphorus and Sulfur (CHNOPS)" are absolutely needed for the formation and survival of every human being, animal & plant. [40-45]
- <u>The size of our Sun is enormous:</u> Our Sun is 864,400 miles (1,391,000 km) across, 109 times our Earth's diameter, weighs about 333,000 times more than our Earth, 93 million miles (149.5 million km) away from our Earth, and our Sun is so humongous that even 1,300,000 Earths could fit inside of it. [61]
- <u>Our Sun has a lifespan of 9 to 10 billion years.</u> Which means our Sun will run out of nuclear fuel, extinguish or die after 4 to 5 billion years. When our Sun dies, our planet Earth, our Moon & 7 other planets will be engulfed with it and possibly vaporized. Afterwards our Sun will either become a white dwarf or explode into a supernova in which case a new star will born out of the debris. [62]
- <u>The water we drink today is at least 4.54 billion years old, older than our planet Earth, older than our Sun, and older than our Solar System</u>. Our planet Earth inherited up to 50% of its water (primordial water) from the interstellar medium even before it was born, and the remaining water came to our planet Earth by the bombardment of Asteroid (not Comets) during and after the early stages of our Solar System formation. Our ancestors' belief that Comets brought water to our planet Earth was later proved by our recent scientists to be a myth! [80-166]

OUR UNIVERSE, OUR STARS, OUR MILKY WAY GALAXY, OUR SOLAR SYSTEM, OUR SUN, OUR PLANET EARTH & OUR MOON: How Were They Created?

FORMATION OF OUR UNIVERSE
BIG-BANG THEORY: A THEORY BASED ON THE SCIENTIFIC FACTS

1. Big Bang Theory: Can We Trust It?

No one knows for sure what triggered the Big Bang. But the discovery of Cosmic Microwave Background radiation in 1965 made the Big Bang theory the best theory of describing the origin and evolution of our Universe. With the aid of the NASA's highly sophisticated spacecraft known as the Wilkinson Microwave Anisotropy Probe (WMAP), ground-based telescopes, and brilliant scientific calculations, our astronomers, cosmologists, space researchers and scientists understood what exactly happened in the beginning stages of our Universe. [22]

● The most important finding was the afterglow of creation, light and radiation leftover from the Big Bang. This relic of the Big Bang pervades our Universe and is visible to microwave detectors as a birthmark, which allowed our scientists to piece together clues of our early Universe. [23, 24, 25]
● This "afterglow of creation" commonly known as the Cosmic Microwave Background radiation is the leftover heat from the fireball of the Big Bang in which our Universe was born 13.8 billion years ago. It provides a unique insight into our Universe's infancy as the world-renowned theoretical physicist and cosmologist late Dr. Stephen Hawking described it as our Universe's "baby photo," and said that it is the discovery of the century if not of all time. And another cosmologist, astrophysicist and Nobel Prize winner Dr. George Smoot said that "it is like seeing the face of the God—the Creator." [26]

After this discovery of the afterglow of creation of our Universe, surrounding light and radiation leftover from the Big Bang, more and more scientists and very many common people around the world started accepting and entrusting the Big Bang theory.

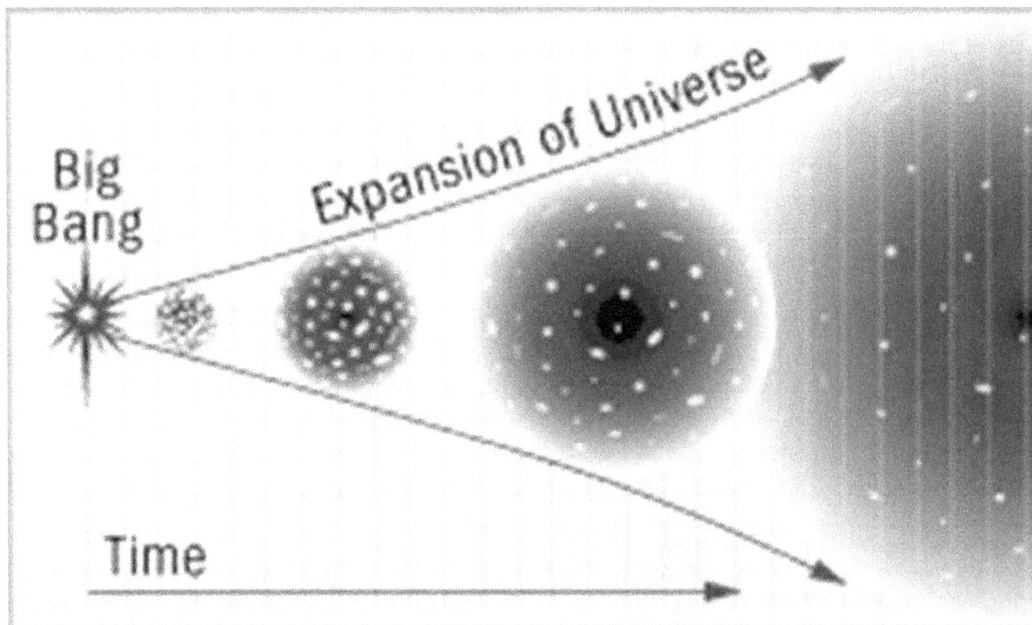

Figure 1.3 Our Universe has begun expanding like a magical balloon immediately after its birth.

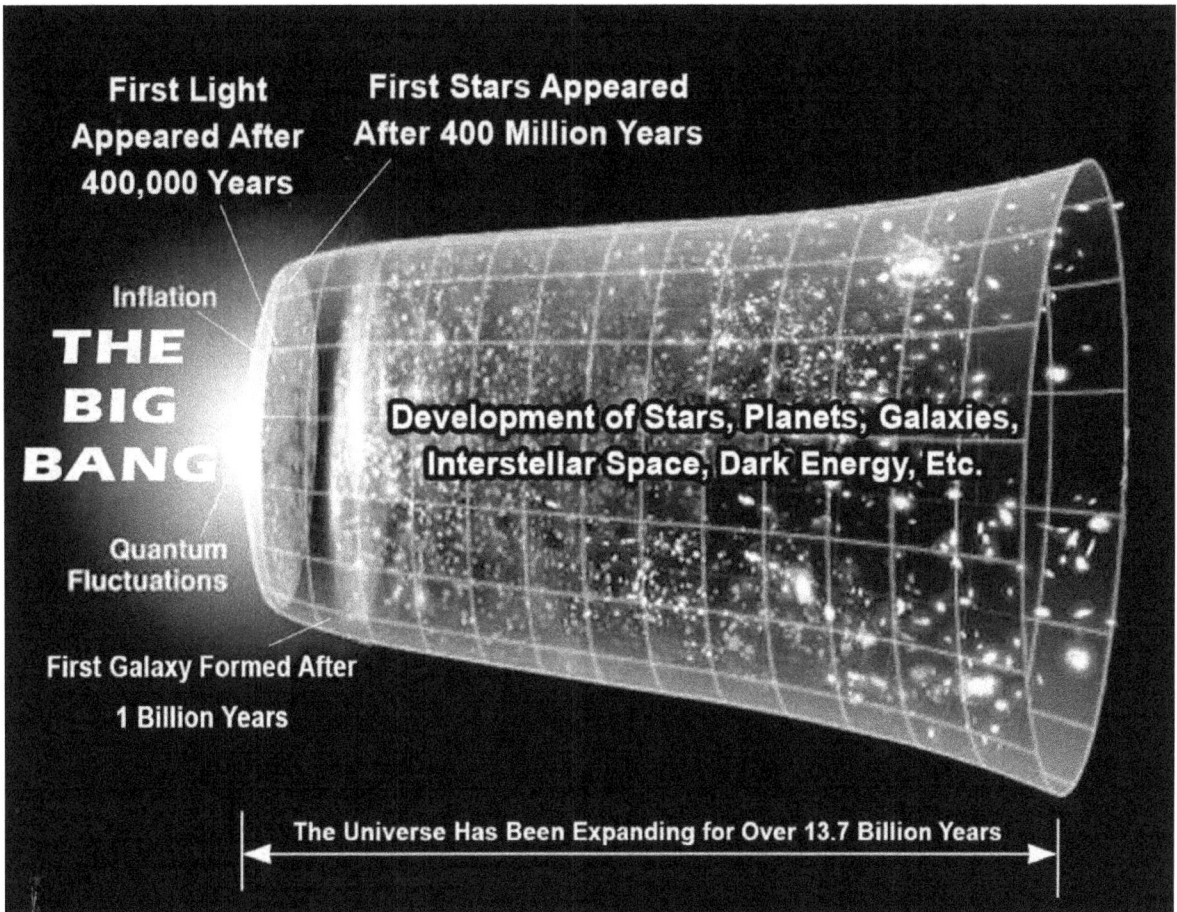

Figure 1.1 The formation of our Universe after the Big Bang.

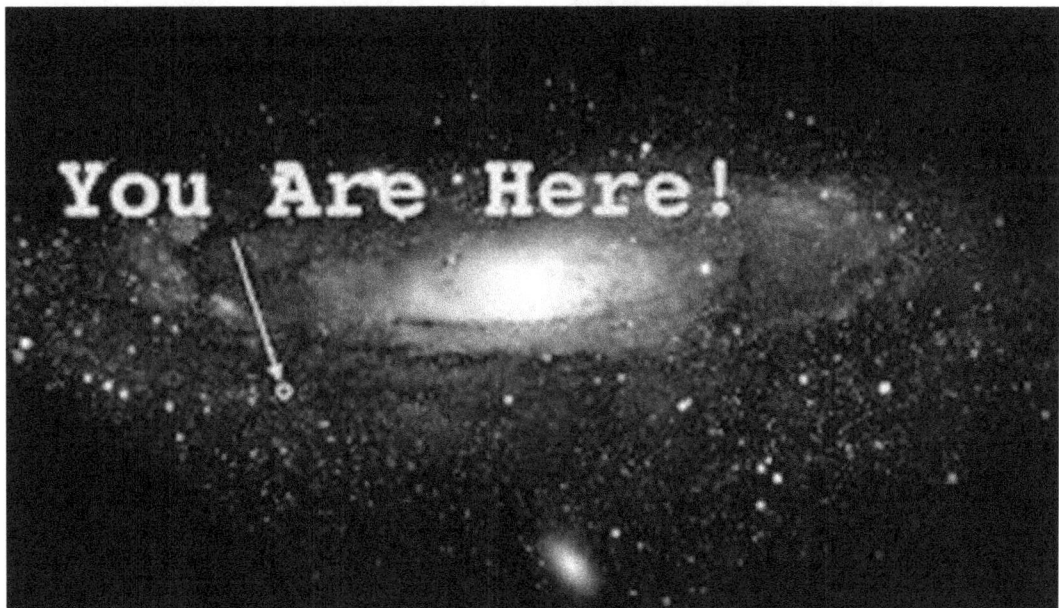

Figure 1.2 Location of our planet Earth on the spiral-shaped Milky Way Galaxy.

2. Big Bang Theory: What Does It Say?

Big Bang theory states that our Universe has begun its formation from an unimaginably hot and dense point of Singularity some13.8 billion years ago, and has started expanding unstoppably since then. The original temperature at the time of birth was infinite or at least 100 Nonillion degrees or 10^{32} degrees Kelvin. [27] When our just-born Universe was unimaginably so young, that is to say when it was only 10^{-34} second young — that is to say, when it was only a hundredth of a billionth of a trillionth of a trillionth of a second in age — Whew!— it underwent an incredible growth spurt or burst of expansion known as inflation in which period the space itself expanded exponentially faster than the speed of light, breaking the laws of physics. *The Big Bang was not a violent explosion, but it was a rapid and peaceful expansion*. During that period of a tiniest fraction of a second, our Universe doubled in size at least 90 or 100 consecutive times, going from a subatomic-sized to the golf-ball-sized instantaneously, and blew up the space like a giant magical balloon into several kilometers, and never stopped expanding thereafter. [23, 27]

3. Big Bang Theory: Singularity, Inflation & Primordial Soup

a. Singularity: A singularity means a point where some property is infinite. If you extrapolate the properties of our Universe to the very instant of the Big Bang, you will find that both the density and the temperature go to infinity. That compacted tiny point with infinite density from which our Universe expanded might have contained all the clues (all the mass, space and time that ever needed), from which the whole Universe emerged. This decision came from the observations of the NASA's WMAP's cosmic microwave background, which contained the afterglow of light and radiation leftover from the Big Bang. [23, 25]

b. Inflation: The initial stage of the Big Bang called "Cosmic Inflation" was so quick, as it lasted only 10^{-34} second. All the energy and heat from that explosion was shot out. And wherever that expansion of that peaceful explosion travelled with time, it automatically created space upon which our Universe lies. [25]

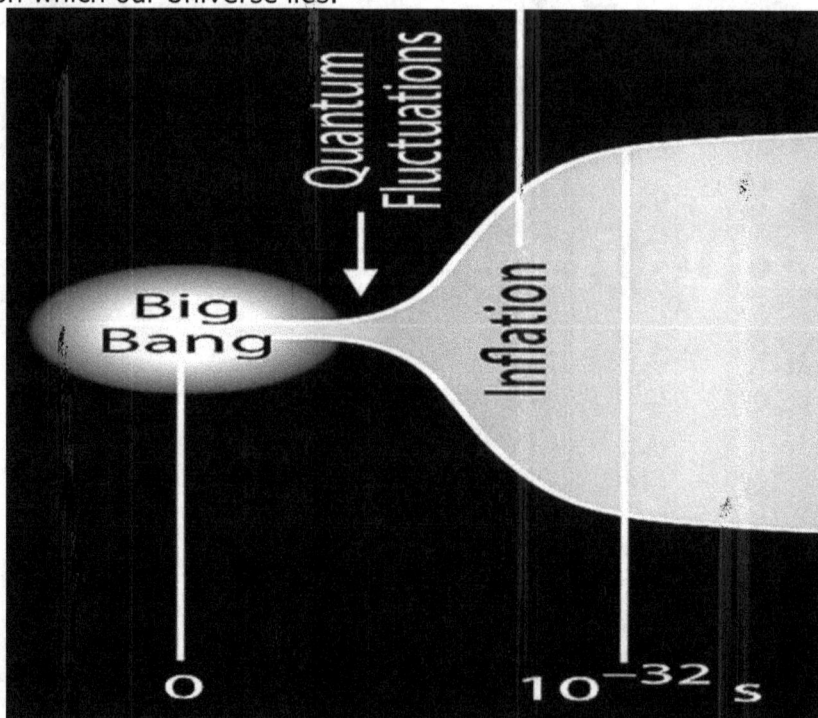

Courtesy of Steemit
Figure 1.4 The inflation ends when time = 10^{-32} second [25]

The temperature of our Universe at that instant was unimaginably 100 Nonillion degrees or 10^{32} degrees Kelvin. [27,28] During that time of Cosmic Inflation, matter and anti-matter annihilated each other, and as a result no matter existed. No atoms were generated yet, even though there was some surplus of quarks left behind. [29]

c. Primordial Soup

Cosmologists believe that our newborn Universe existed as a hot and dense primordial soup, broth or plasma of highly energized matter, went through a burst of expansion like a giant magical balloon faster than the speed of light. At that incredibly high temperature and high pressure, matter was crushed into a soup of its constituent quarks, electrons and gluons (no atoms were formed yet). Our just-born Universe was found to be doubled its size at least 90 consecutive times in a span of 10^{-32} second. This phase of primordial soup, also known as **Cosmic Inflation**, ended when our Universe was only 10^{-32} second old. [25]

● Everything in our Universe, including every person in this world, is made up of atoms. Science tells us that those atoms consist of nuclear particles called protons and neutrons in their hearts. These subatomic particles, in turn, are made up of building blocks known as quarks, which are glued together by particles aptly named gluons. [18] However, during the time of Inflation, our Universe was so hot that quarks were kept apart from gluons. The result would have been a hot dense mixture of quarks and gluons known as a quark-gluon plasma. During that state of primordial soup, atoms were not yet created, but all the matter existed in a special state of baryons (protons and neutrons), and at that instant our Universe was extended into only a few kilometers across. [30]

d. Our Scientists Have Recreated the Big Bang's Primordial Soup Conditions, and Achieved a Temperature of 5.5 Trillion °K in A Giant Atom Smasher at CERN'S Large Hardon Collider!

CERN (Conseil Européen pour la Recherche Nucléaire), Geneva, Switzerland:[30, 31, 32, 33]

It is the European Organization for Nuclear Research, also called CERN in French language, that operates the largest particle physics laboratory in the world. On August 13, 2012, the scientists at CERN's Large Hadron Collider (LHC), Geneva, Switzerland, announced that they had achieved temperatures of over 5 trillion °K and perhaps as high as 5.5 trillion °K when they attempted to recreate the conditions of the Big Bang's "Primordial Soup" that represented the earliest moments following the Big Bang.
The giant 27 kilometer (16.7 mile) long particle accelerator is the most powerful in the world, and only it can generate the appalling energies needed to probe these earliest conditions of our Universe. The research team had been using the ALICE (A Large Ion Collider Experiment) experiment to smash together "lead ions" at 99% of the speed of light (Speed of light is 186,000 miles per second or about 300,000 Kilometers per second) to recreate a quark-gluon plasma – an exotic state of matter (Primordial Soup) believed to have filled our Universe just after the Big Bang during the time of inflation. The accelerator slammed the lead nuclei together at a record energy level of 5.02 tera electron Volts (TeV), or about 5 trillion electron Volts. When the nuclei collided at a slightly off center angle, they formed a football-shaped "droplet" of quark-gluon plasma as shown in the figure below. The whole scientific community marvelled by this groundbreaking achievement.

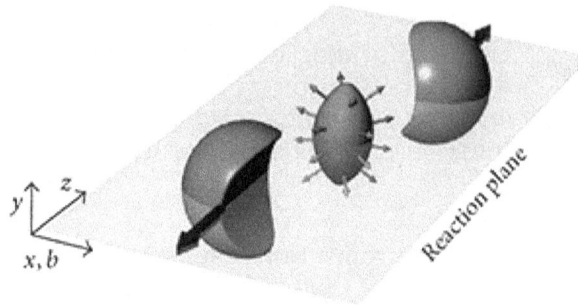

Courtesy of the University of Copenhagen, Denmark.
Figure 1.5 The formation of football-shaped quark-gluon plasma was recorded.
A temperature from 5 trillion °K to 5.5 trillion °K was also recorded.

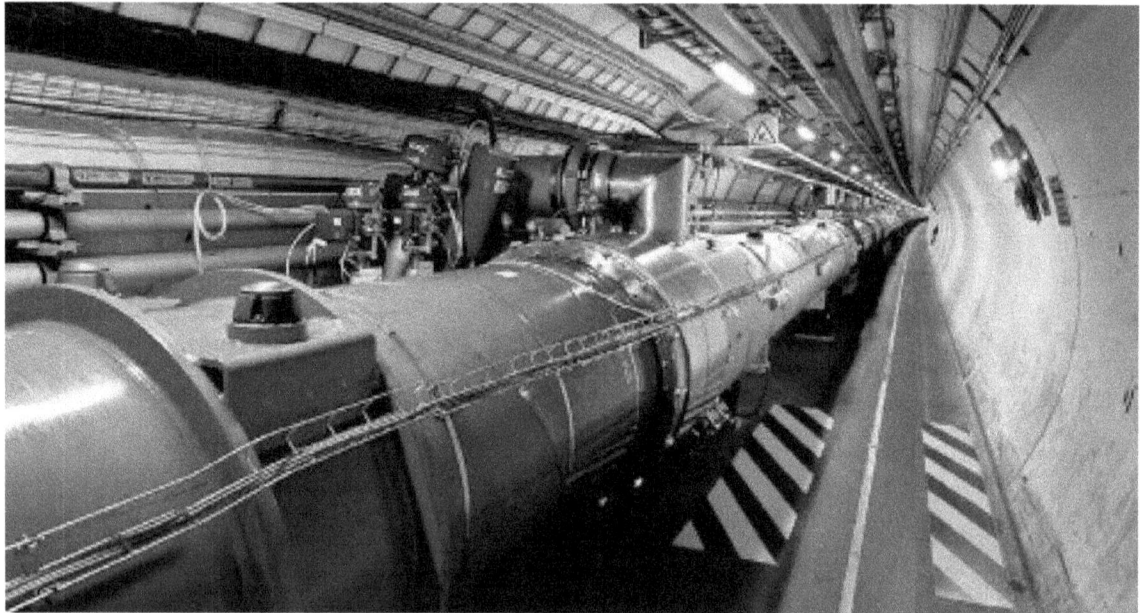

Courtesy of CERN, Geneva, Switzerland
Figure 1.6 Large Hardon Collider (LHC), Recreation of Early Universe, CERN, Geneva, Switzerland.
The giant 27 kilometer (16.7 mile) long particle accelerator.

4. Nearly One Second After the Big Bang, Our Universe Has Cooled Down, Temperature Dropped to 1 Billion Degrees Kelvin,
and the most fundamental particles such as quarks, electrons, photons and neutrinos just formed, but not yet bound together. [27, 28, 33]

⊛ Our Universe continued to expand not as quickly as during inflation, but at a much slower rate. As our Universe was further being cooled down and expanded, it was being governed by the four fundamental forces such as:
(i) the gravity,
(ii) the strong force,
(iii) the weak force, and
(iv) the electromagnetic force.

5. Nearly 3 Minutes After the Big Bang, The First Most Important Event Took Place: Hydrogen & Helium Nuclei Were Created!

Our Universe was still unimaginably hot, but there was an exponential drop in temperature. The temperature of our Universe dropped from 100 Nonillion degrees or 10^{32} degrees Kelvin to 1 billion degrees Kelvin or 10^9 degrees Kelvin. That sudden drop in temperature caused a kind of cooling effect as the energy solidified into matter. That cooling process is analogous to the way how steam condenses to liquid droplets as water vapor cools in steam distillation, or how the water is being frozen into ice in the freezer [34, 35]. Those cooling conditions (both temperature and pressure) of our newborn Universe 3 minutes after the Big Bang perfectly suited for the quarks to coalesce and bound into hadrons such as protons and neutrons. It was called hadrons era. The protons and neutrons in turn combined to form nuclei of light elements such as hydrogen and helium. No neutral atoms were created yet. That was the first most important event that took place in the history of the Big Bang because:

Our visible Universe today is approximately composed of: [35]
  ▹ 90% Hydrogen (by mole fraction),
  ▹ 8% Helium (by mole fraction), and
  ▹ 2% Everything Else (by mole fraction).

6. Nearly 380,000 Years After the Big Bang, The Second Most Important Event Took Place:

The primary element "Hydrogen" was created, and thereafter hydrogen was abundantly available throughout our Universe. The nuclei of the light elements such as hydrogen, helium, lithium and beryllium attracted electrons, and formed neutral or stable atoms in a process known as "stellar nucleosynthesis."   The First Light Appeared! { **LET THERE BE LIGHT!** }

During 300,000 to 380,000 years after the Big Bang, our Universe was still unbearably too hot for light to shine. Nearly 380,000 years after the Big Bang, the temperature of our Universe dropped to about 4000 degrees Kelvin, and then to 3000 degrees Kelvin. [36]

◉ RECOMBINATION PERIOD: [29, 37]

REMEMBER! About 3 minutes after the Big Bang, the quarks coalesced and bound into hadrons such as protons and neutrons. The protons and neutrons in turn combined to form nuclei of light elements such as hydrogen and helium. About 380,000 years after the Big Bang, our Universe was filled with a hot and dense fog of ionized gas. The nuclei of the light elements **hydrogen, helium, lithium and beryllium** attracted electrons, and formed neutral and stable atoms in a process called "**nucleosynthesis**". Hydrogen is the dominant primordial element created 380,000 years after the Big Bang, as our scientists now know that 90% of the Universe today is made made up of hydrogen. This process of particles pairing up in order to form stable atoms was called "Recombination", and that process actually started occurring approximately 240,000 to 300,000 years after the Big Bang, and intensified after 380,000 years. Our Universe went from being opaque to transparent at this point. Up to 300,000 years after the Big Bang, light had formerly been stopped from traveling freely because it would frequently scatter off the free electrons. About 380,000 years after the Big Bang, the free electrons were bound to protons in an attempt to form neutral atoms, and therefore the light was no longer being impeded. Even though our Universe became transparent relatively, our Universe at that point of time was not fully visible because THERE WERE NO STARS.

FORMATION OF STARS

7. Nearly 400 Million Years After the Big Bang, The Third Most Important Event Took Place:

The First Stars Appeared, and the Formation of Stars and Planets Continued Until Today!

Nearly 400 Million Years After the Big Bang, our Universe already switched to cold weather, below freezing temperatures. The temperature dropped to and varied between − 213 °C and -254 °C (between 60 °K and 19 °K). [29]

◔ REIONIZATION PERIOD [27, 29, 37]

● Some Big Bang theorists believe that the first stars began their formation 200 million years after the Big Bang, but some other scientists believe that the first stars were clearly visible after 400 million years. However, NASA posted that there was no documented evidence with regard to when exactly the first stars began to form.

About 400 Million years after the Big Bang, our Universe emerged out of darkness. This period in our Universe's evolution is called the age of "Reionization" in which period <u>clumps of gas consisting of large coulds of all sorts of neutral atoms of many elements produced during the "Recombination Process," collapsed under gravity with internal spinning and swirling to form the very first bright light, which became a star,</u> thereby creating the first <u>star, and followed by more and more stars, which led to building the very first Solar System</u>, and eventually millions of stars along with orbiting planets (Solar Systems). The emitted ultraviolet light from these energetic events cleared out and destroyed most of the surrounding neutral hydrogen gas. The process of reionization plus the clearing of foggy hydrogen gas caused our Universe to become transparent to ultraviolet light for the first time. This dynamic phase of formation of stars and galaxies lasted over 500 million (half a billion) years, and the reionization process lasted about 1 billion years. The first galaxy was formed about 1 billion years after the Big Bang. [27]

FORMATION OF STARS, GALAXIES, CLUSTERS & SUPER CLUSTERS

The early stars were made up of very simple and light gaseous elements (hydrogen and helium) and so they had very short lifespans of only millions of years. But the nuclear fusion in the cores' of these early stars slowly created all kinds of heavier elements, including the most important carbon and oxygen. When a large star died, it would become a part of a new star in the supernova explosion. In the beginning, these stars were created in small groups and attracted other stars. These stars were grouped in irregular shapes. Then the different shapes merged to form the first galaxies. Then as more and more galaxies formed, they were grouped in galaxy clusters, and then these clusters were contained in super clusters. Today, our scientists know about a force called dark energy. Dark energy acts like an anti-gravity and does the opposite of gravity. Dark energy is currently the cause of the expansion of our Universe. Our Universe is expanding at an accelerating rate today. With the discovery of dark energy, many scientists now believe that our Universe will continue to expand forever and all of the matter in our Universe will eventually decay in about one trillion years. [38]

<u>**How Many Stars Are There in Our Universe?**</u> Dr. RK Has Made the Following Calculation:

Our Universe is embedded with 2 trillion galaxies = 2×10^{12} galaxies.

Our Milky Way Galaxy has 500 billion stars = (1/2) trillion stars = $(1/2)(10^{12})$ stars

Therefore Total Number of Stars = $(2 \times 10^{12})(1/2)(10^{12}) = 10^{24}$ stars = Trillion Trillion stars.

There are 1,000,000,000,000,000,000,000,000 stars. There are 10^{24} stars.

That's a 1 followed by twenty-four zeros.

This is a grossly rough estimate. The exact number of stars is unknown.

COUNTING STARS IN THE SKY OF OUR UNIVERSE [6, 18]
METHOD 1

Counting stars in the sky of our Universe is like trying to count the number of sand grains on a beach. We might be able to calculate the surface area of the beach by measuring the length and width of the beach by means of a measuring tape, and we can also measure the depth of the sand grains spread all over the beach by means of a measuring tape, and then we could calculate the volume of the total sand grains on the beach in cubic centimeters (cm^3) by using the formula "volume of the total sand grains a beach = length x width x depth". Supposing that each sand grain is a spherical particle, and by measuring the radius of a grain in centimeters, we can calculate the volume of each sand grain in cubic centimeters (cm^3) by using the formula $(4/3)\,\pi\,r^3$ where r is the radius of the sand grain (a spherical particle). If we divide the volume of the total sand grains of the beach by the volume of each sand grain, we obtain the total number of sand grains in that beach by simple math. This is just a simple example that can be understood by any person with a high school background. Our astronomers in the past used to apply this kind of simple technique in determining the number of stars in our Universe by visual observation using a telescope. The more experience an astronomer has, the more accurate the star-count could be. [6]

Counting stars in the sky of our Universe is always a grossly rough estimate (Even the NASA does not know total stars) as it is impossible to count the stars accurately. Over time, the space research progressed a lot. On space, astronomers wouldn't try to count stars individually, instead they measure integrated quantities like the number and luminosity of galaxies. ESA's infrared space observatory Herschel has made an important contribution by 'counting' galaxies in the infrared, and measuring their luminosity in this range. From these experiments, they found the number of galaxies in our Universe. By multiplying the number of galaxies in our Universe by the number stars in each galaxy, they were able to determine the total number of stars. [6]

For Example, A ESA's Astronomer Has Made The Following Calculations: [6]

For Example, A ESA's Astronomer Has Made The Following Calculations: [6]
Suppose that our Universe has 10^{11} to 10^{12} Galaxies.
Each Galaxy has has 10^{11} to 10^{12} Stars.
Total number of Stars in our Universe (grossly rough estimate) = 10^{22} to 10^{24} Stars.

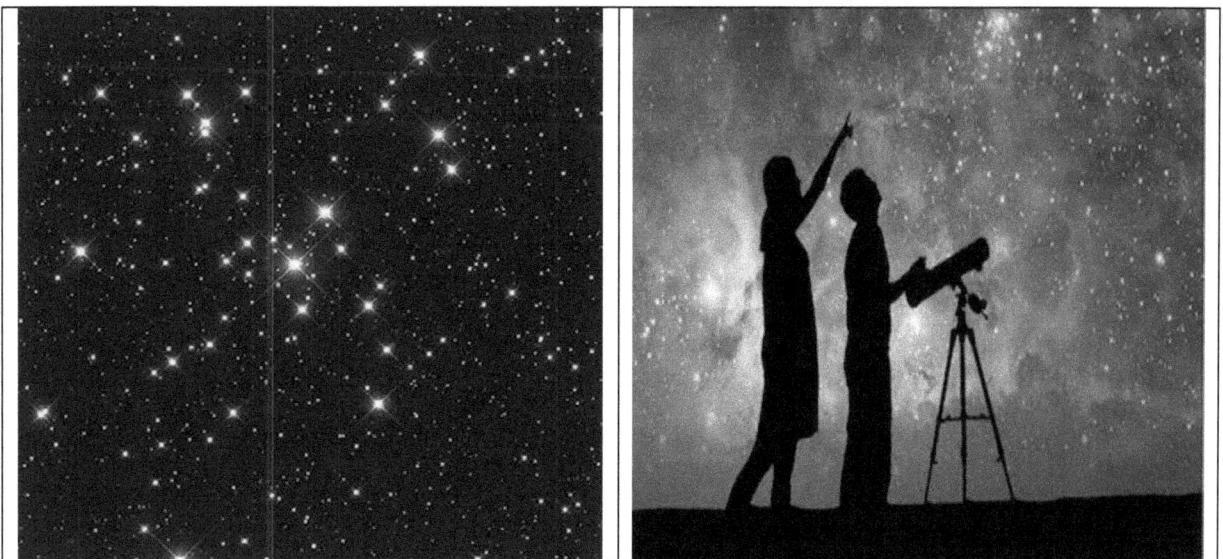

Figure 1.7 Counting stars in the sky of our Universe.
Counting stars in the sky by visual observation by our astronomers is believed to be an art.

METHOD 2

The primary way astronomers estimate stars in a galaxy is by determining the galaxy's mass. The mass is estimated by looking at how the galaxy rotates, as well as its spectrum using spectroscopy. Once a galaxy's mass is determined, the other tricky thing is figuring out how much of that mass is made of stars. Most of the mass will be made up of dark matter, a type of matter that emits no light but which is believed to make up most of the mass of our Universe. You have to model the galaxy and see if you can understand what percentage of that mass of stars would be. If we can determine mass of the galaxy and the mass of the interstellar space, we can calculate the total mass occupied by stars. By supposing an average mass for each star (Of course, not all stars have equal mass), we can approximately compute the total number of stars in a galaxy. In a typical galaxy, if you measure its mass by looking at the rotation curve, about 90 percent of that is dark matter. [18]

Much of the remaining "stuff" in the galaxy is made up of diffused gas and dust. A scientist estimated that about 3 percent of the galaxy's mass will be made up of stars, but that could vary. Further, the size of the stars itself can greatly vary from something that is the size of our sun, to something dozens of times smaller or bigger. So is there any way to figure out how many stars are for sure? In the end, it comes down to a rough estimate only. In one calculation, the Milky Way has a mass of about 100 billion solar masses, so it is easiest to translate that to 100 billion stars (In general a galaxy is believed to have one trillion stars). This accounts for the stars that would be bigger or smaller than our Sun, and averages them out. However, the mass is tough to calculate. More sophisticated instruments are being manufactured to determine the mass of a galaxy. By multiplying the number of galaxies discovered by the number of stars in each galaxy, our scientists determine the rough estimate of number of stars in our Universe. [18]

Stars Manufacture Heavier Elements Like Factories Do! [39, 40, 41]

RECAP: The nuclei of the primordial elements "hydrogen and helium" were created 3 minutes after the Big Bang. Nearly 380,000 years after the Big Bang, when the first light appeared, the nuclei of the light elements attracted electrons, and formed neutral atoms. Which means the actual stable atoms of the light elements "hydrogen, helium, lithium & beryllium" were created at the time of recombination in a process called nucleosynthesis well before the stars formation. Nearly 400 million years after the Big Bang, the primitive (first) stars formed as clumps of gas (mostly hydrogen) collapsed enough under gravity to form the very first bright light, which became a star, thereby creating the first star, followed by more and more stars, and eventually millions of stars, billions of stars, and even trilions of stars. Hydrogen is the primordial element created 380,000 years after the Big Bang, and is used as the burning fuel in the stars. Hydrogen is never created or produced in stars. But all the other heavier elements are produced in the burning cores of stars 400 million years after the Big Bang. [39]

● Stellar Nucleosynthesis: When a gigantic interstellar cloud of space dust and primordial gas (mostly hydrogen) is collapsed due to gravity, a protostar forms and proceeds to compact further. The protostar becomes a disk and starts rotating, spinning and swirling under gravity. The rotation of the protostar (the disk) helps preventing further collapse, but internal spinning and swirling continues within the cloud, forming much stronger protostar. The continuing gravitational compaction causes the protostar to heat up more and more until its core reaches a critical temperature of about 15,700,000 °C. At this extremely high temperature, hydrogen atoms are disassociated into protons and electrons, as they no longer bound together. When the temperature in the burning star rises to 15 million to 100 million degrees Celsius, the dissociated protons and electrons are brought back together by a fundamental force called "strong nuclear force", thereby creating a much heavier element called helium. This process in which a heavier element is created in the burning cores of stars is called nuclear fusion or stellar nucleosynthesis. Then the helium star lights up and shines again. [40]

Stellar Nucleosynthesis (Continued)

Stellar Nucleosynthesis is a process in which heavier elements are created within a star by combining the protons and neutrons together from the nuclei of lighter elements at extremely high temperatures (millions of degrees) when stars run out of fuel, extinguish or die, and then explode into supernovae.

Supernova explosion occurs in a galaxy when a huge star runs out of nuclear fuel (hydrogen or helium), collapses and explodes while manufacturing, dumping and scattering all kinds of heavier elements into the interstellar medium, from a gigantic cloud of which a typical Solar System is created.

Primitive stars were massive, short-lived, collapsed under gravity, and exploded into supernovae while manufacturing all kinds of heavier elements. Hydrogen was the primary element from which all heavier elements were created in the following manner: [41]

- **Hydrogen** was first fused to produce helium in the burning core of a star or stars.
- Helium in turn was fused to produce lithium.
- Lithium plus helium in turn was fused to produce beryllium.
- Beryllium plus helium in turn was fused to produce **carbon** (very important element).
- Carbon plus helium was fused to produce **nitrogen** (very important element).
- Carbon/Nitrogen plus helium was fused to produce **oxygen** (very important element).
- Oxygen plus helium was fused to produce neon.
- Neon plus helium was fused to produce magnesium.
- Magnesium plus helium was fused produce silicon.
- Silicon plus helium was fused to produce **sulfur** (very important element).
- Sulfur plus helium was fused produced argon.
   Sulfur was also produced from silicon via an alpha process.
- **Phosphorus** was produced via neutron capture onto isotopes of silicon (very important).
- Argon plus helium was fused to produce calcium.
- Calcium plus helium was fused to produce titanium.
- Titanium plus helium was fused to produce chromium.
- Chromium plus helium was fused to produce iron.

Similarly all those 117 heavier elements of our periodic table were manufactured in the burning cores of stars.

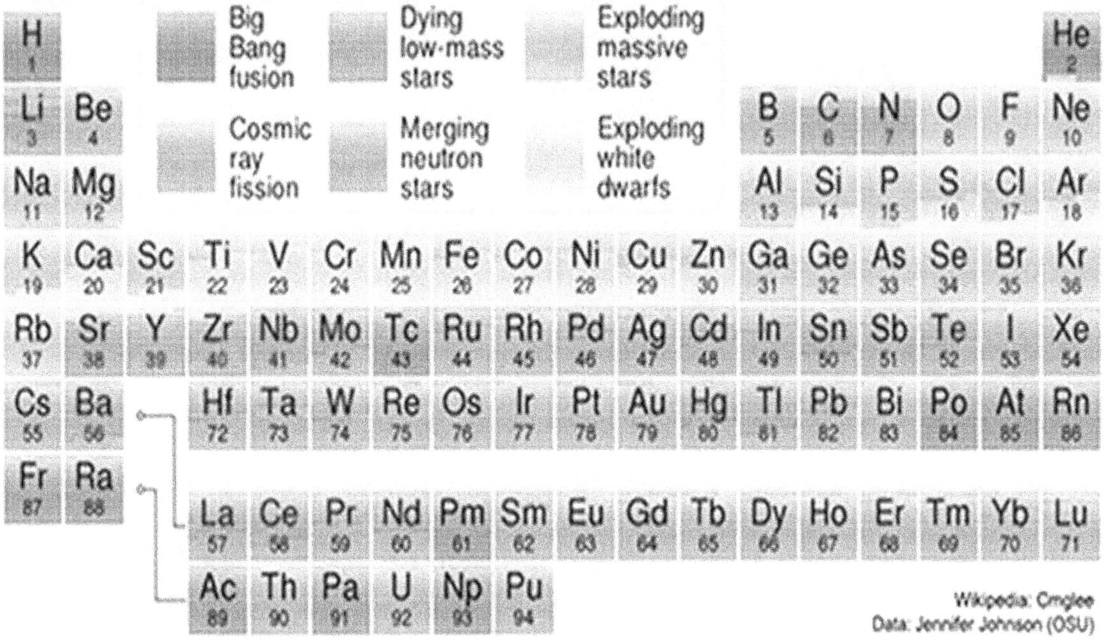

Courtesy of Nasa Science (Nasa.gov) and Wikipedia: Cmglee

Figure 1.8 Periodic Table (All these heavier elements were manufactured in the burning cores of stars).

● In the stellar nucleosynthesis, many different reactions take place in many different ways in the interiors of collapsing stars. It is called the triple-alpha process in which helium-4 nuclei (alpha particles) are transformed to produce the next heavier element. Each heavier element is produced when a star reaches a distinct core temperature (sometimes, tens of millions of degrees), heat and radiation. Sometimes the catalytic chemical reaction also takes place.

● Early stars were massive, short-lived and exploded into supernovae while manufacturing, dumping and scattering all those 117 heavier elements (except hydrogen) of our periodic table into the interstellar space from a gigantic cloud of which our Solar System was created!

● Did you know? When our solar system began its formation 6 billion years ago from a gigantic cloud of space dust and interstellar gas, that gigantic cloud was already enriched with all those 117 elements, and that is how our planet Earth possessed all those 117 heavier elements.

IMPORTANT NOTE: NASA's scientists, astronomers & space researchers studied extensively the possibility of the formation and existence of life in the other planets of our Solar Sytem, and always adopted that "Life requires 6 essential elements such as CHNOPS: carbon, hydrogen, nitrogen, oxygen, phosphorus and sulfur." [42, 43]

WHEN YOU LOOK UP AT NIGHT, YOU ARE SEEING FACTORIES CALLED STARS

When you look up at night, you are seeing factories called stars equipped with nuclear-fusion reactors, working round the clock, without which the constituents for our entire natural world would not exist, including all those 117 heavier elements of our periodic table desperately needed for the formation and survival of every human being, animal & plant. [40]

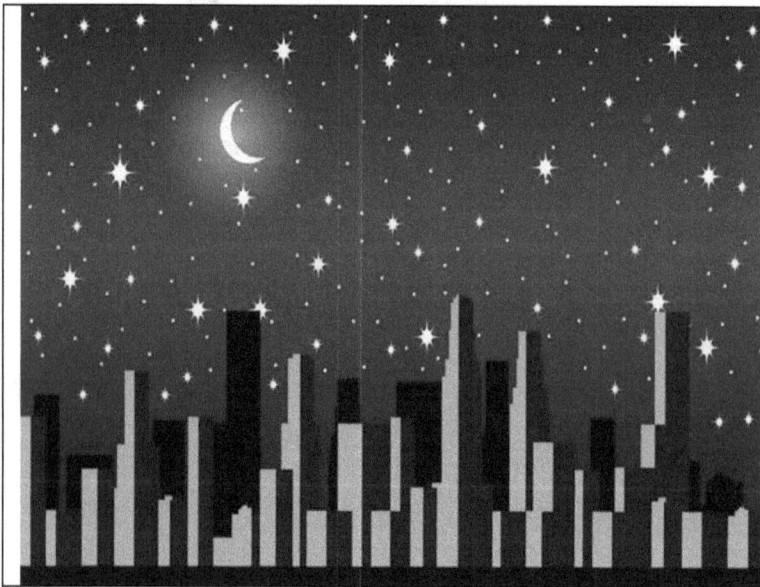

Astronomer Dr. Carl Sagan in his book "Cosmos" wrote: The nitrogen in our DNA, the calcium in our teeth, the iron in our blood, the carbon in our apple pies were all made in the interiors of collapsing stars. We are all made of starstuff. [44]

Almost 99% of the mass of the human body is made up of SIX elements "carbon, hydrogen, nitrogen, oxygen, phosphorus and sulfur." And the remaining 1% is made up of other elements. All organic matter containing carbon was produced originally in the stars. [45]

Figure 1.9 When you look up at night, you are seeing factories called stars.

The Process of Stars Creation Continued Until Today!

The process of stars creation continued, as our Universe has begun creating millions of stars along with orbiting planets and galaxies, and then billions of stars along with orbiting planets and galaxies, and then even trillions of stars along with orbiting planets and galaxies that are visible today!

The Current Temperature of Our Universe in the Year 2020

The current temperature of our Universe in 2020 = −270.42 °Celsius = 2.73 °Kelvin. [36]

FORMATION OF OUR MILKY WAY GALAXY

In general our Universe has 3 types of galaxies (there are 2 trillion galaxies): [46]
(i) Spiral-shaped galaxy
(ii) Elliptical-shaped galaxy
(iii) Irregular-shaped galaxy

❧ **Milky Way Galaxy:** Please see Figure 1.2. We live on a planet called "Earth" that is a very small part of our solar system, manufactured by our Sun. But our solar system itself is a tiny portion of our Milky Way Galaxy, which is again a tiny portion of our unimaginably humongous Universe that has been expanding unlimitedly for 13. 8 billion years. A galaxy is a huge collection of gas, dust, and of billions or trillions of stars and their solar systems. A galaxy is held together by gravity.

❧ Our Milky Way Galaxy is spiral-shaped upon which we all live, and our solar system (our Sun, our Earth & other 7 planets, our Moon) formed on one of the spiral arms as shown in the figure below. Astronomers now believe that our Milky Way Galaxy is approximately 13.6 billion years old. [11]

❧ Just like our planet Earth goes around the Sun, the Sun goes around the center of the Milky Way Galaxy. It takes one year or 365 days for our planet Earth to go around our Sun, and it takes 250 million years for our Sun and our entire solar system to go all the way around the center of our Milky Way Galaxy. [19]

❧ Our Milky Way Galaxy has 100 billion stars (solar systems) on the lower end and 400 billion stars (solar systems) on the upper end, totaling 500 billion solar systems. Our solar system (our Sun, our planet Earth, 7 other planets and our Moon) is one of them. Inside the Milky Way Galaxy, most stars have at least one planet orbiting the solar system. However, there are many stars without planets orbiting.

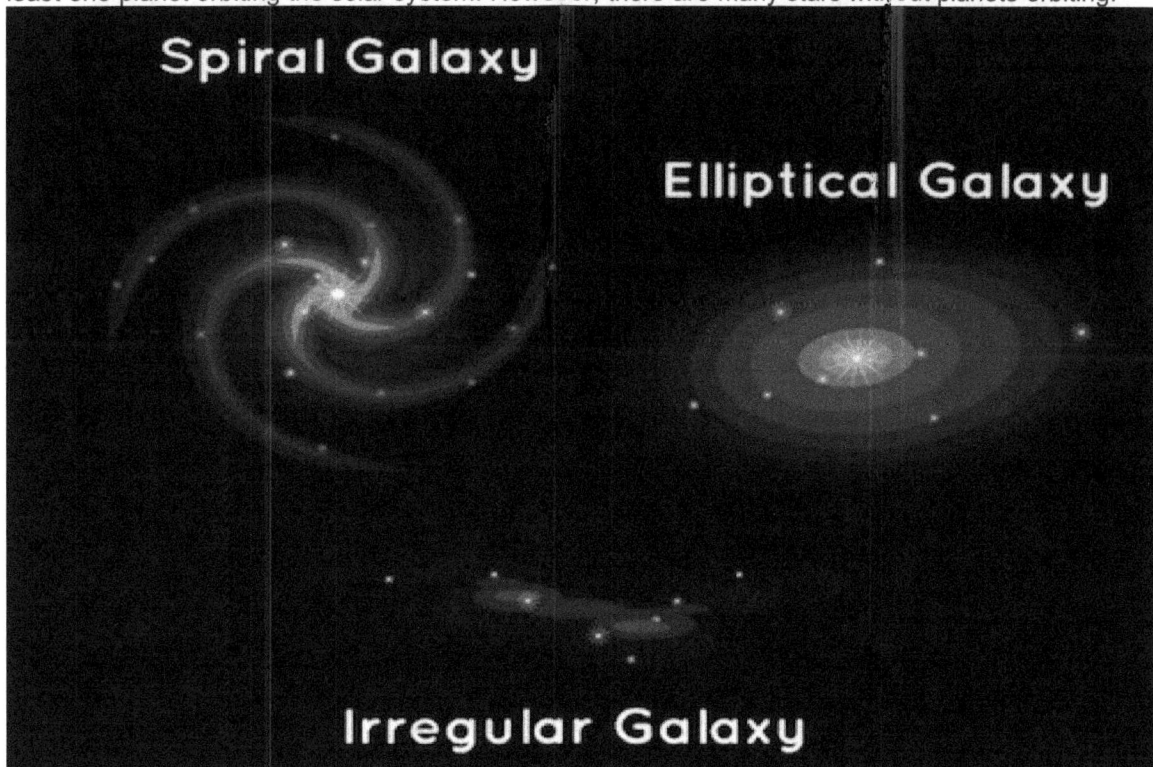

Spiral Galaxy

Elliptical Galaxy

Irregular Galaxy

Courtesy of Nasa.gov

Figure 1.10 Galaxies are spiral-shaped, elliptical-shaped, oval-shaped or irregular-shaped. [46]
Milky Way Galaxy is spiral-shaped upon which we all live. Please see Figure 1.2.

● **BLACK HOLE:** Our Milky Way Galaxy has a supermassive black hole, filled with dark energy, in the middle of it. [46]   A black hole is a region of space exhibiting extremely strong gravitational acceleration. In black holes, no particles or even electromagnetic radiation such as light can pass through or escape from. The strong gravity occurs because matter has been compressed into a tiny space. This compression can take place at the end of a star's life when it runs out of fuel. Some black holes are a result of dying stars.

● **Why Was It Called Milky Way Galaxy?** At first the Greeks and then the Romans called it "Milky Way" because if you look upward, either with your naked eye or by means of a telescope, on a clear night from the Earth's darkest regions, you could glimpse a broad stripe of stars, cloaked in clouds of dust and gas, arching across sky, and it would make you feel that you are witnessing a **milky patch**. The Milky Way Galaxy was found to glow in the night sky over the Chile's La Silla Observatory, La Higuera, Coquimbo Region, Chile, South America. [47, 48]

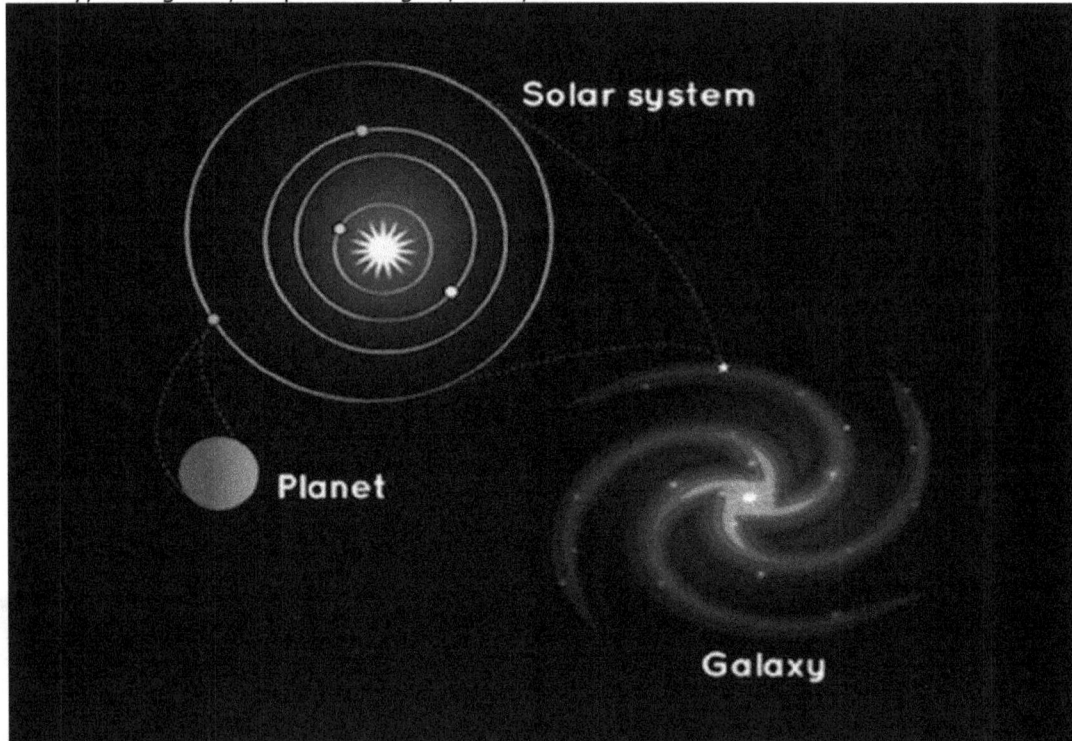

Courtesy of Nasa.gov

Figure 1.11   Our Milky Way Galaxy is spiral-shaped, and our Solar System formed on one of the spiral arms. [46]

LIGHT-YEAR | NEAREST STAR | NEAREST GALAXY

LIGHT-YEAR: A light-year is not time, but a light-year is a unit of distance. It is the distance that light can travel in one year. Light travels at a speed of 186,000 miles per second or 300,000 km per second. So in one year, light can travel about 10 trillion km. More precisely, one light-year is equal to 9,500,000,000,000 kilometers. The distance between stars in our galaxy and in our Universe is so vast that astronomers and scientists cannot indicate it in kilometers or miles, but rather express it in light-years.
● Our Milky Way Galaxy is about 150,000 light-years across.

NEAREST STAR: Alpha Centauri is nearest star, much larger star than our Sun. It is 4.3 light-years away. Our scientists believe that for humans to travel to the nearest star, it would take at least 70,000 years.

NEAREST GALAXY: Andromeda Galaxy is the nearest spiral galaxy, much larger than our Milky Way Galaxy, and is approximately 2.5 million light-years away. Our Milky Way Galaxy as a whole is moving through space at a rate of approximately 600 km per second and our scientists believe that it will collide with the Andromeda Galaxy in about 4 billion years. By that time our Sun could be exhausted, running out of fuel, extinguishing and about to collapse and explode into supernova. [12]

FORMATION OF OUR SOLAR SYSTEM [55, 56, 57, 58, 59, 60]
OUR SUN, OUR PLANET EARTH, 7 OTHER PLANETS, OUR MOON, ASTEROIDS, COMETS, Etc.
Did You Know Our Sun Manufactured Our Solar System?

Astronomers, space researchers and scientists figured out that a Solar System, consisting of a star and several planets that orbit the star, is created from the supernova explosion of a deceased star.

WHAT IS A SUPERNOVA? Supernova explosion occurs in a galaxy when an enormously large star (10 to 20 times larger than our Sun) runs out of nuclear fuel (hydrogen and/or helium), and when some of its mass flows into its core, and the core collapses as it cannot withstand its own gravitational force. Supernovae have been observed by our astronomers as monster explosions in galaxies. Larger stars have shortened lifespan as they need more fuel to burn whereas relatively smaller stars have longer lifespan as they need less fuel to burn. When a massive star runs out of nuclear fuel, it will be collapsed as it cannot withstand its own gravitational force, and explodes into a supernova while manufacturing, dumping and scattering heavier elements into the interstellar space from a gigantic cloud of which, a Solar System is created.

WHAT IS A SOLAR NEBULA? [55, 56]

☻ A gigantic interstellar cloud known as "solar nebula" of space dust (cosmic dust) and space gas that was squeezed by a supernova explosion gave birth to our solar system. A nebula is nothing but a huge cloud of interstellar gas and space dust mixed and coalesced with the leftovers of a previous star upon death. Each cloud of an extinguished or deceased previous star is capable of generating dozens of stars in a galaxy, though some stars are larger than the others.

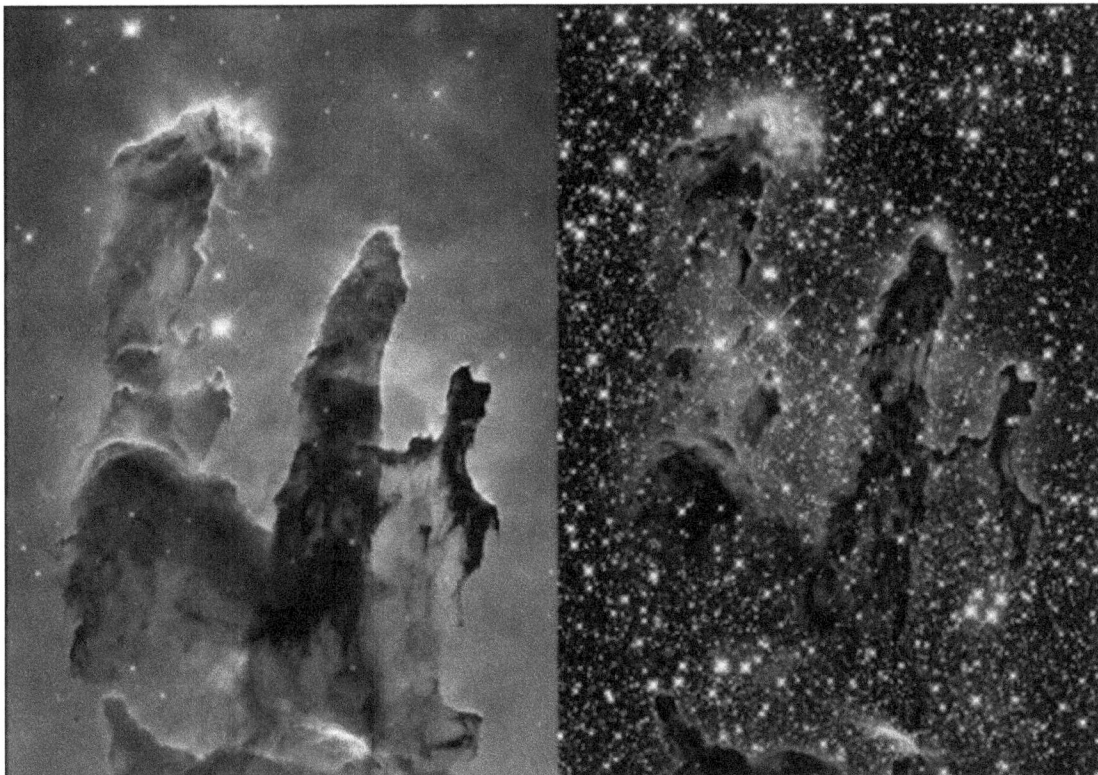

Courtesy of Nasa.gov   **Pillars of Creation**

Figure 1.12 A solar nebula is a gigantic cloud of space dust & gas of a deceased star.

⊕ According to the Big Bang theory, our solar system began its formation some 6 billion years ago. By that time, the stardust in the space and interstellar gas were already enriched abundantly with all kinds of elements. There are 118 all kinds of elements listed in our periodic table such as hydrogen, helium, lithium, carbon, oxygen, nitrogen, calcium, iron, phosphorous, iodine, magnesium, zinc, selenium, copper, manganese, chromium, molybdenum, chloride, and many other components. All these elements (except hydrogen) were manufactured in the burning cores of earlier stars.

⊕ **Please Refer to Figure 1.13:** A gigantic interstellar cloud known as "solar nebula" of space dust and primordial gas that was squeezed by a supernova explosion gave birth to our solar system. A nebula is nothing but a huge cloud of interstellar gas and space dust that was already enriched with all kinds of heavier elements, mixed, coalesced and squeezed together with the leftovers of a previous star upon death. The giant interstellar cloud collapsed under gravity and began rotating, compacting, spinning and swirling for 100s of millions of years or even billions of years, until our solar system formed! Our solar system began its formation some 6 billion years ago. Our scientists estimated that the age of our Earth and therefore the age of our solar system is 4.54 billion years, which means it took some one and half billion years to complete our solar system formation.

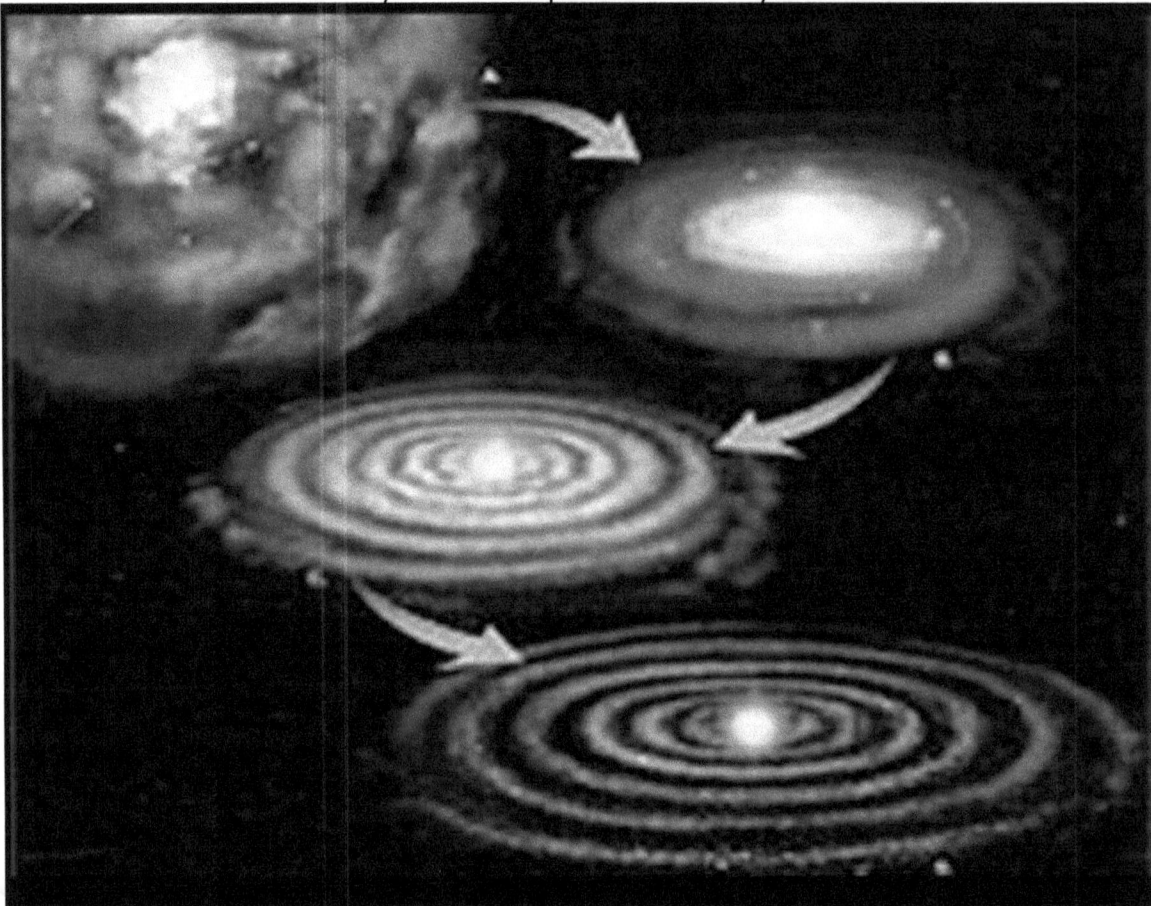

Figure 1.13 Our Solar System was being formed from a solar nebula.
A nebula is nothing but a gigantic cloud of interstellar gas and space dust.

⊕ Experts believe that more than 99% of the gigantic interstellar cloud of the space dust and the interstellar gas, from which our solar system was being developed, becomes the Sun, and the remaining portion (less than 1%) becomes the planets that orbit the Sun for 100s of millions of years, or even billions of years before the solar system is completed its formation.

● **Please Refer to Figure 1.14:** Upon the collapse of the gigantic cloud of space dust and primordial gas (mostly hydrogen), a protostar formed and proceeded to compact further. The protostar became a disk and started rotating under gravity. The rotation of the protostar (the disk) helped preventing further collapse, but internal spinning and swirling continued within the cloud, forming much stronger protostar. The central core reached a balance between the gravitational force and the internal pressure, aka as hydrostatic equilibrium, after 100s of millions of years. The rotation of the disk helped preventing further collapse of the disk, but internal spinning and swirling continued within the cloud, forming the protoplanetary disk.

● Just like a dancer that spins faster as she pulls in her arms, the cloud began to spin as it collapsed. Eventually, the cloud grew hotter and denser in the center, with a disk of gas and dust surrounding it that was hot in the center but cool at the edges. As the disk got thinner and thinner, particles began to stick together and form clumps. Some clumps got bigger, as particles and small clumps stuck to them, eventually forming 8 planets, their moons, asteroids, comets, meteorites, near-earth objects, etc.[60]

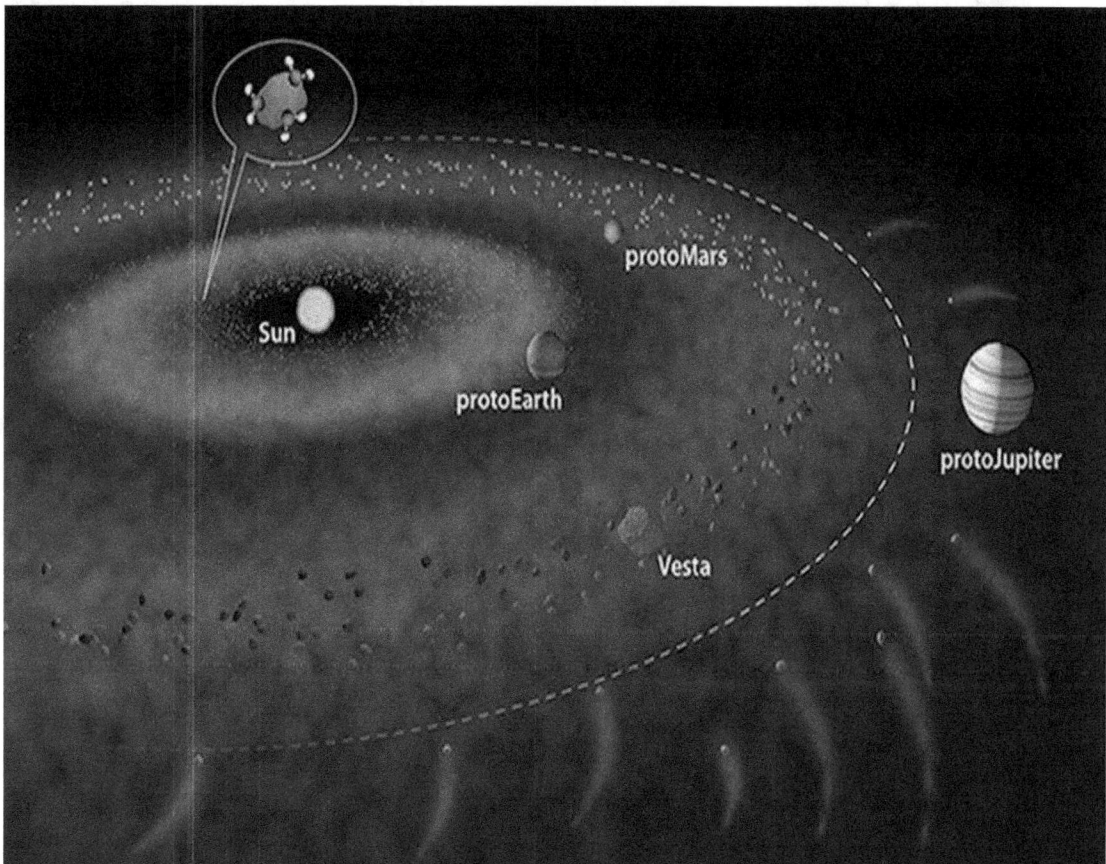

Courtesy of Jack Cook, Woods Hole Oceanographic Institution.
Figure 1.14 Our Solar System formation (Protoplanetary disks).
ProtoEarth, ProtoMars, ProtoJupiter = The planets that are at an early stage of development.
The Protostar (our Sun) was actually being orbited by 8 Protoplanets (some of them were not yet formed).
A protostar is a very young star that is still gathering mass from its parent molecular cloud. A protoplanetary disk or a protoplanet is a rotating circumstellar disk of dense gas and dust surrounding a young newly formed star.

SUMMARY: A gigantic cloud of space dust and interstellar gas of the supernova explosion of a massive, collapsing, exploding, spinning and swirling deceased star gave birth to our Solar System. That gigantic cloud was already enriched with all those minerals that we use today to remineralize and alkalize the purified water. That gigantic cloud was also already filled with liquid water. And that is how our planet Earth possessed that much liquid water that we drink to survive today.

FORMATION OF OUR PLANET EARTH [57, 58, 59, 60]

⊕ This process of spinning, swirling and the accretion in the solar system continued for 100s of million of years, or even billions of years, until the larger solid balls of accretion completed, and gave birth to 8 planets, including our planet Earth. It took more than a billion years for the formation of our solar system including all 8 planets, their moons, asteroids, comets, near-earth objects, etc.

Please Refer to Figure 1.15: Near the center of the burning Sun where only rocky material could stand the great heat, the four terrestrial or inner planets "**Mercury, Venus, Earth and Mars**" formed. And away from the centre of the burning Sun or farther to the burning Sun, icy and gassy matter settled in the outer regions of the disk, where the other four giant or jovian outer planets "**Jupiter, Saturn, Uranus and Neptune**" formed as shown in the figure below.

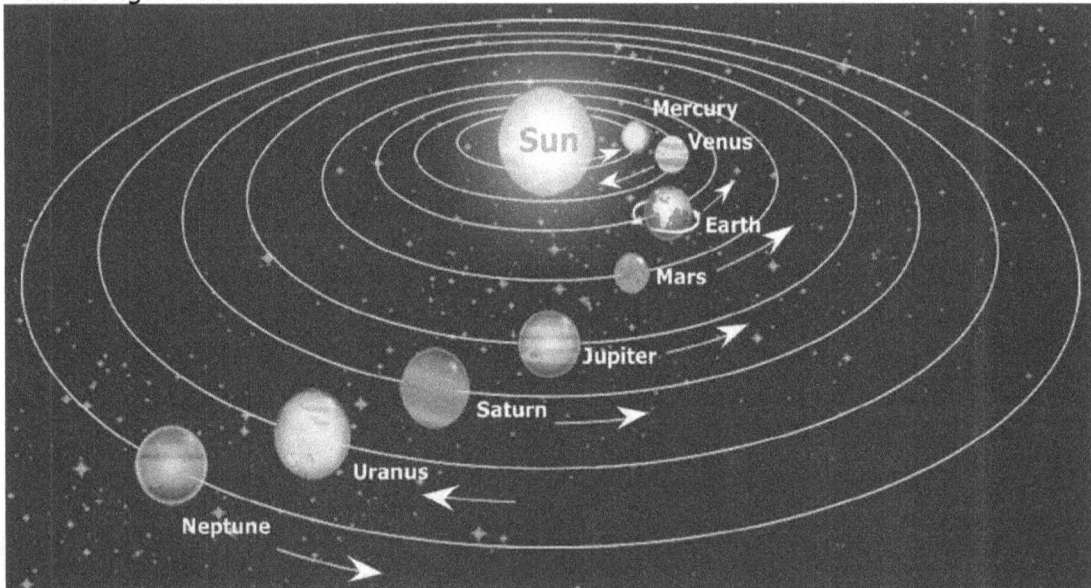

Figure 1.15 Formation of our solar system along with 8 planets, including the Earth.

⊕ Our Sun manufactured our solar system, including our planet Earth, as the process of spinning and swirling of a gigantic cloud of the space dust and the interstellar gas continued for one and half billion years! Our Sun is now being orbited by 8 planets named "Mercury, Venus, Earth, Mars, Jupiter, Saturn, Uranus and Neptune". Our solar system began its formation 6 billion years, and completed its formation 4.54 billion years ago. In the next half a billion years, our planet Earth is going to be accompanied by our Moon (read below).

⊕ **The Size of our Sun is Enormous:** Our Sun is 864,400 miles (1,391,000 kilometers) across, 109 times the Earth's diameter, weighs about 333,000 times more than Earth, 93 million miles (149.5 million km) away from Earth, [61b, 61c] and our Sun is so humongous that even 1,300,000 Earths could fit inside of it. [61]

⊕ **How Long Our Sun Lasts?** Our Sun has a lifespan of 9 to 10 billion years. Which means our Sun will run out of nuclear fuel, extinguish or die after 4 to 5 billion years. When our Sun dies, our planet Earth, our Moon and 7 other planets will be engulfed with it and possibly vaporized. Afterwards our Sun either will become a White Dwarf or will explode into a supernova in which case a new star will born out of the debris. [62]

FORMATION OF OUR MOON [63, 64]

● Our solar system began its formation some 6 billion years ago. The formation of our planet Earth and other 7 planets completed 4.54 billion years ago. After our terrestrial planet Earth was solidifying from its lava, softer elements moved to the surface and harder elements moved to the center of the core of our Earth. Some 4 Billion years ago, suddenly a large object (a meteorite) of the size of the mars smashed on to the surface of our Earth, creating a huge blast. Our planet Earth swallowed up much of the object's particles, ejecting a huge beam of dust and particles on to its atmosphere. These particles of debris gathered together and formed a much smaller planet-like object called Moon. Thus our Moon was formed. The formation of our Moon was an incredibly important event in the history of our Earth, especially in the development of life.

● The size of our Moon (equivalent to the size of Mars) perfectly suited our planet Earth, and gave stability to the development of our planet Earth and to the Earth's axis. Our Moon's gravitational force and at the same time its attachment to our planet Earth protected our planet Earth from wabbling while rotating on its own axis and orbiting around our Sun. Our Moon also helped our Earth's rotation by slowing down a little thereby establishing smooth rotation. Our planet Earth, at the time of its birth, was actually rotating so fast that it took only 6 hours to complete one rotation per day. After the formation of our Moon, our Earth's rotation stabilized and started completing one rotation in 24 hours, thereby creating the day-and-night cycle for us.

● Our Moon also provided our Earth the very important seasons "spring, summer, autumn and winter" in sequence, which are very important for the plants to grow and life to occur and to survive on our planet Earth.

● Our Moon and the presence of the plenty of liquid water in our planet Earth were both greatly responsible for the formation and development of life on our planet Earth.

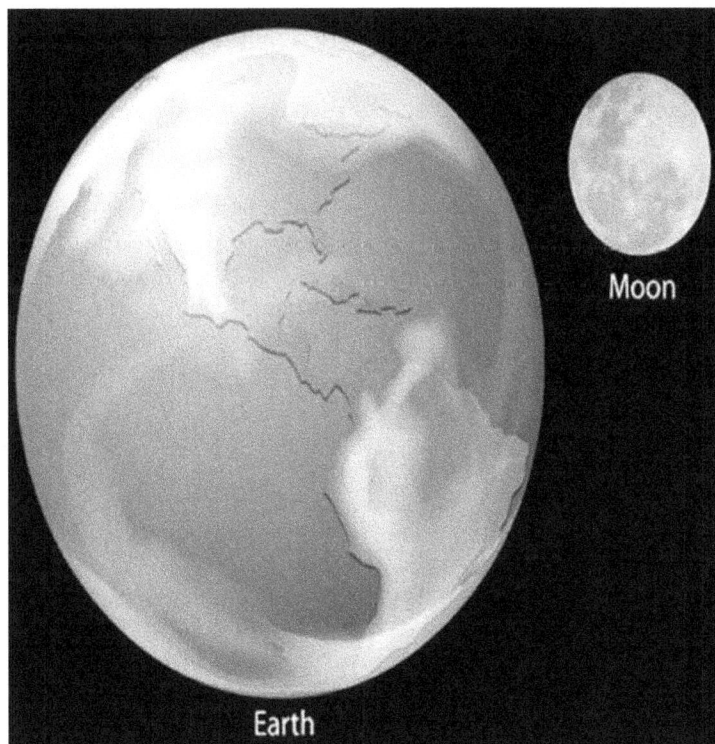

Figure 1.16 Formation of our Moon occurred 4 billion years ago, and gave stability to our Earth's rotation.

FORMATION OF OUR PLANET EARTH & MOON (Continued)

Our Earth at the time of its birth was rotating so fast to complete one rotation per day. After the attachment of our Moon, Earth's rotation slowed down, stabilized, and started completing one rotation in exactly 24 hours. We now know that the Earth, by rotating around its own axis and by orbiting (revolving) around the Sun, creates day and night. It now takes 24 hours for our Earth to complete one rotation around its own axis (12 hours for the day and 12 hours for the night). It takes precisely 365 ¼ days (1 year) for our Earth to orbit, revolve or circle around the Sun.

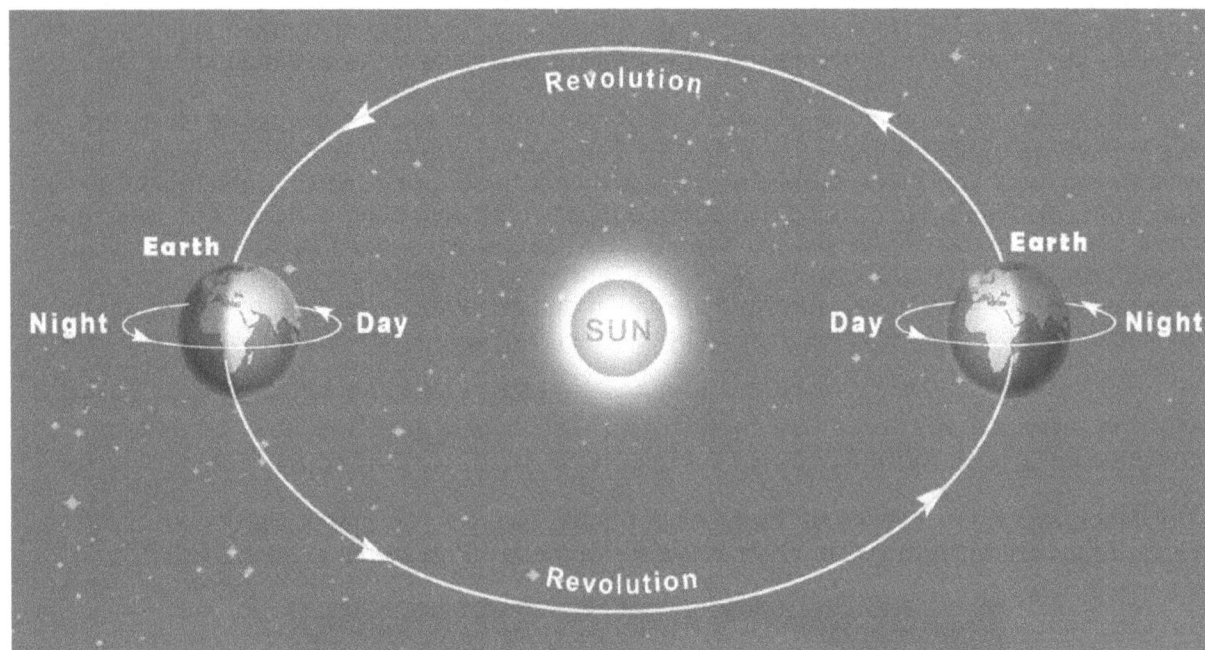

Figure 1.17 Our Earth, by rotating on its own axis and by revolving around the Sun, creates day & night. It takes 24 hours to complete one rotation, and our Earth revolves around our Sun in 365 ¼ days (1 year).

FORMATION OF ASTEROIDS, COMETS AND METEORITES

Asteroids, comets, moons, meteors, meteorites and many other near-Earth objects are now understood to be the leftover debris from the formation of the solar system. Astronomers and scientists around the world currently think that our solar system's 8 planets (Mercury, Venus, Earth, Mars, Jupiter, Saturn, Uranus and Neptune) and minor bodies, including asteroids, comets, moons, meteorites and many other near-Earth objects all formed from the same cloud of stardust and gas of the supernova explosion of a collapsing massive star. Asteroids & comets cannot be considered as planets because they are relatively small in size.

Asteroids are rocky fragments that orbit the Sun in a belt between Mars and Jupiter. Scientists think that there are probably millions of asteroids, ranging widely in size from less than one kilometer wide to hundreds of kilometers across. The asteroid belt is located between Mars and Jupiter. Scientists believe that stray asteroids or fragments from earlier collisions have slammed into our planet Earth in the past, and played a major role in the evolution of our planet Earth. Researchers also determined that ice-bearing asteroids brought water, life-forming substances and other useful elements to the Earth during the period of their bombardment in the early stages of the formation of our planet Earth. Which means our planet Earth by the time of its formation already possessed liquid water. Researchers now have scientific evidence that our planet Earth attained 50% of its water from the bombardment of Asteroids.

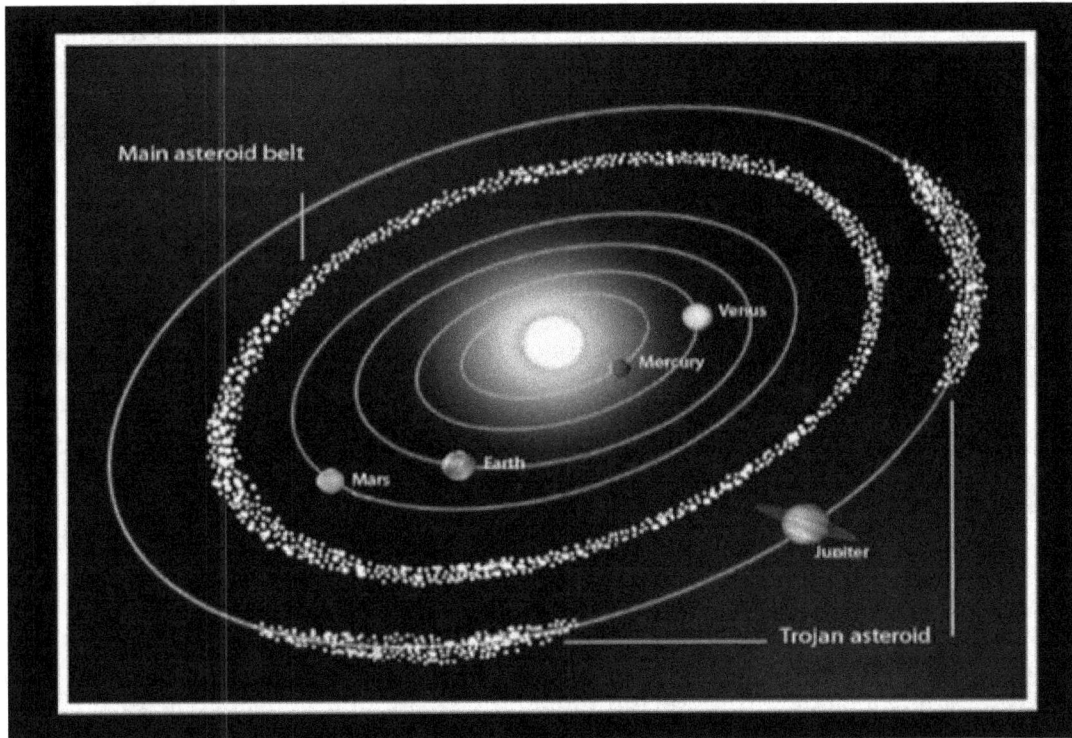

Figure 1.18 The asteroid belt is between Mars and Jupiter.

AGE OF OUR UNIVERSE & OUR MILKY WAY GALAXY [1, 2, 3, 4, 5, 11, 12, 13]

The Hubble Space Telescope, launched in 1990, has helped our astronomers tremendously to measure the age of our Universe. Our astronomers have figured out several ways of observing and determining the age of our Universe.

(i) By measuring the speeds and distances of galaxies, our astronomers determined the age of our Universe. Because all of the galaxies in our Universe are generally moving apart, we infer that they must all have been much closer together sometime in the past (since our Universe has been created, it has been expanding all the time). Knowing the current speeds and distances to galaxies, coupled with the rate at which our Universe is being accelerated, it became possible to calculate how long it took for them to reach their current locations. The answer was about 13 to 14 billion years repeatedly.

(ii) The second method involves measuring the ages of the oldest star clusters. Globular star clusters orbiting our Milky Way are the oldest objects our astronomers found and a detailed analysis of those stars revealed that they formed about 13 to 14 billion years ago. The good agreement between the above-mentioned two very different methods is an encouraging sign that our space scientists are in the right track.

(iii) The Wilkinson Microwave Anisotropy Probe (WMAP), originally known as the Microwave Anisotropy Probe (MAP), is a NASA Explorer mission that launched in June 2001 to make fundamental measurements of cosmology, the study of the properties of our Universe as a whole. Headed by Professor Charles L. Bennett of Johns Hopkins University, the mission was developed in a joint partnership between the NASA Goddard Space Flight Center and Princeton University. WMAP has been stunningly successful, producing our new Standard Model of Cosmology. WMAP's data stream has ended. In 2012, NASA's Wilkinson Microwave Anisotropy Probe (WMAP), after collecting a vast amount of data for over a period of 9 years, estimated the age of our Universe to be 13.772 billion years, with an uncertainty of plus or minus 59 million years. Therefore,

The age of our Universe = 13.8 Billion Years.   **Please see Figure 1.1.**

Some astronomers and scientists believe that first stars appeared after 200 million years, and others believe after 400 billion years. So the Milky Way began its formation 200 to 400 million years after the Big Bang. Therefore,

The age of our Milky Way Galaxy = 13.4 to 13.6 Billion years. Please see Figure 1.2.

AGE OF OUR PLANET EARTH BY RADIOMETRIC DATING [65-71]

● The age of our planet Earth was determined by radiometric dating, which is the most accurate and reliable method to date old rocks. The nuclei of radioactive elements decay or spontaneously break down at predictable rates. For example, half of a given batch of uranium will decay into lead every 710 million to 4.47 billion years, depending on the isotope used (this number is termed the element's "half-life"). That uranium, which was created during a supernova that occurred long before our solar system existed, lingers in trace amounts within the Earth. When a rock is formed in the bowels of the planet, uranium atoms are trapped within it. These atoms will decay as the rock ages, and by measuring the ratio of radioactive isotopes within the rock, scientists can figure out how long it has been around. [66]

● The oldest rocks on Earth, found to date, are the Acasta Gneiss in northwestern Canada near the Great Slave Lake, which are 4.03 billion years old. But rocks older than 3.5 billion years can be found on all continents. Greenland boasts the Isua supracrustal rocks (3.7 to 3.8 billion years old), while rocks in Swaziland are 3.4 billion to 3.5 billion years. Samples in Western Australia run 3.4 billion to 3.6 billion years old. The age of a zircon crystal from Australia was found to be 4.4 billion years, and is the oldest piece of Earth yet found (after our scientists believed the rock of Acasta Gneiss in northwestern Canada is the oldest). Our scientists have collected and calculated the ages of some 70 meteorites that have fallen from sky on to the Earth by using the radiometric dating technique. The oldest of these rocks are reported to be between 4.4 billion and 4.5 billion years old. [67]

● An age of 4.55 ± 0.07 billion years, very close to today's accepted age, was determined by Clair Cameron Patterson using uranium-lead isotope dating (specifically lead-lead dating) on several meteorites including the Canyon Diablo meteorite and published in 1956. [70]

● In 1972, Apollo 17 mission brought back the oldest Moon rocks of our solar system ever collected and archived thus far have the radiometric dates of up to 4.54 billion years. [68]

▷ The age of our planet Earth, our Sun & our Solar System is therefore 4.54 Billion years.

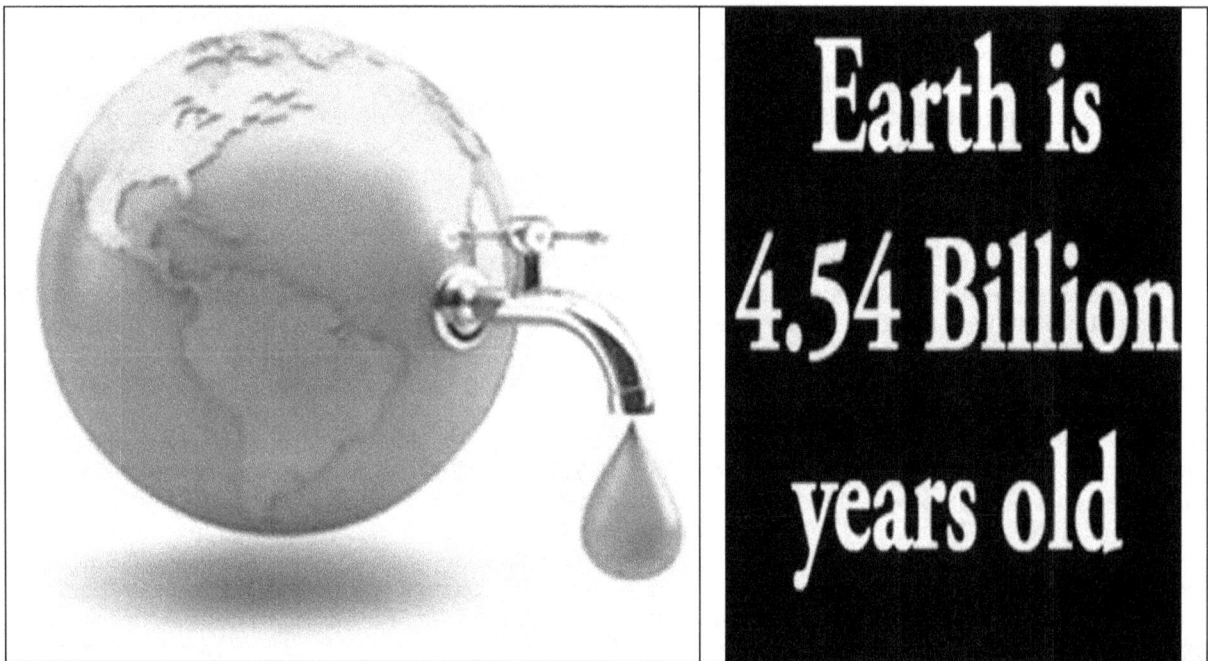

Figure 1.19 Our Planet Earth was manufactured by our Sun 4.54 billion years ago, and was getting ready to harbor life. Our planet Earth, our Sun and our Solar System were all formed at the same time, 4.54 billion years ago.

Age of Our Planet Earth and Our Sun

◉ Based on the aforementioned scientific evidence on age determination of diverse ancient rocks by radiometric dating technique of our Earth and Moon, our scientists have confirmed that the age of our planet Earth (and therefore our Sun and all items in our Solar System) as 4.54 billion years. This most updated estimate is being endorsed by the NASA (National Aeronautics and Space Administration), Washington D.C., USA, and many other space agencies around the world.

◉ Our Sun has a total lifespan of 9 to 10 billion years. Our Sun will extinguish or die after 4 to 5 billion years. When our Sun dies, our planet Earth and other 7 planets will be engulfed with it.

About Our Planet Earth [72-75]

◉ Our planet Earth is the third rotating and revolving planet from the Sun, and is the only astronomical object known to harbor life. Based on the radiometric dating and other sources of evidence, astronomers and scientists confirmed and verified that our planet Earth is 4.54 billion years old. So far it is the most accurate measurement or calculation of our Earth's age by highly experienced scientists. This age has been endorsed by NASA and other space agencies around the world.

◉ Our planet Earth has a surface area of approximately 510 million square kilometers or 196.9 million square miles. [72, 73]

◉ Our planet Earth as a matter of fact is the only green planet in our Solar System, besides its blue color from the space because of its dominant oceans. Our planet Earth has life or biosphere, possessing vast lengths of free land, oceans, plenty of water, and stable atmosphere to breathe in and breathe out oxygen.

◉ Our planet Earth's natural resources include air, water, soil, minerals, fuels, plants and animals. Our planet Earth has become the homeland to all forms of life such as humans, animals, plants, vegetation, fishes, birds, microbes, many forms of organisms, and so on.

◉ Our planet Earth is naturally equipped to recycle all the matter within it, as is highly capable to turn the waste into treasure and makes itself habitable instantly, no matter how much garbage the people throw in it. Much of what is considered a waste is reused in a closed system where matter is always locked in.

◉ By the year 2017, our planet Earth has become the homeland for more than 7.6 billion human beings.[74]

Water On Our Planet Earth [74, 75]

◉ Liquid water, in addition to oxygen, is the principal ingredient necessary for the formation of life and for human body survival on our planet Earth. Without water, we wouldn't have been here on the planet Earth!

◉ Liquid water is a universal solvent and a mediator of life's chemical reactions, and is the most essential ingredient for the kind of delicate chemistry that helps the formation of life. Water is beneficial and vital to the life of every human being, animal and plant. Did you know more than 99% of an adult body's molecules are water molecules, and 55% to 60% of the adult human body weight is water?

◉ Liquid water on our planet Earth is very abundant. About 71 percent of our Earth's surface is covered by liquid water. According to NASA's report, there are more than 326 million trillion gallons of liquid water on our Earth. [76]

◉ Our Earth's oceans contain about 96.5 percent of all the planet's liquid water. Less than 3 percent of all liquid water on our Earth is freshwater, easily accessible and usable for drinking. More than two-thirds of our Earth's freshwater is locked up in ice caps and glaciers. [75, 76]

Population On Our Planet Earth [74]

◉ The world population was 7.6 billion in 2017, and is expected to reach 8.6 billion in 2030, 9.8 billion in 2050 and a staggering 11.2 billion in 2100, according to a new United Nations report. Our planet Earth is capable to accommodate all kinds of life forms, no matter how high the world's population growth is (unless a catastrophic incident or incidents may occur).

WATER FORMATION ON OUR PLANET EARTH (5 THEORIES)? [80-166]

The puzzling question on everyone's mind is: **"How did the Earth possess that much water (more than 326 million trillion gallons)?"** Astronomers, space researchers, scientists and very many academic researchers have been struggling to find out the truth throughout the human history, but were unable to come up with a definitive answer thus far. However all those scientific research findings can be summarized into the following 5 theories. These 5 theories are discussed in detail along with journal publications in Chapter 20.

THEORIES OF WATER FORMATION ON OUR EARTH	CONCLUSION
1. COMETS COULD HAVE BROUGHT WATER TO EARTH ● Our Solar System (Our Sun, Our Earth and other 7 Planets) began its formation 6 billion years ago, and completed its formation 4.54 billion years ago. Our ancestors believed that ice-bearing comets probably bombarded our Earth 4 to 3.8 billion years ago, and brought water to Earth. This theory is now believed to be wrong because (D/H Ratio) of the water from comets is much higher than that of ocean water. Our ancestors' belief that comets brought water to our planet Earth was however proved by our most recent scientists to be a myth.	MYTH!
2. ASTEROIDS (METEORITES /CARBONACEOUS CHONDRITES) COULD HAVE BROUGHT WATER TO EARTH ● Water-rich asteroids (meteorites / carbonaceous chondrites) impacted the infant Earth about 4 to 3.8 billion years ago, distributing water across the planet by brute force. As a result, our oceans formed. This theory is more accurate because D/H Ratio of the water from asteroids matched well with that of ocean water. Research proved that our planet Earth attained up to 50% of its water from the asteroids during the early stages after the formation of our Solar System.	TRUE!
3. EARTH INHERITED ITS WATER FROM THE INTERSTELLAR MEDIUM ● Water is known to form in the clouds of gas and dust of the interstellar medium (ISM). Our Solar System was created 6 billion years ago from a gigantic cloud of interstellar gas and stardust. That cloud collapsed and formed a solar nebula—a spinning, swirling disk of material under gravity. Scientists found that the primordial water of the interstellar medium survived within the particles of the stardust, and carried forward all the way until and after the formation our Earth. Researchers concluded, from an extensive experimental study and mathematical modelling, that our planet Earth inherited up to 50% of its water from the interstellar medium even before our Solar System was created. Our Solar System completed its formation 4.54 billion years ago. However the water we drink today is at least 4.54 billion years old.	TRUE!
4. EARTH'S DEEP MANTLE HAS THE PRIMORDIAL WATER FROM THE INTERSTELLAR MEDIUM ● The researchers collected samples of primitive rocks from the Baffin Island, Nunavut Territory, Canada back in 1985. Water analysis revealed that these rocks have lower amount of deuterium, and lower D/H Ratio, indicating that the Earth's deep mantle attained the primordial water from the interstellar medium. Which means the water we drink today is at least 4.54 billion years old.	TRUE!
5. THICK HYDROGEN LAYER COULD HAVE REACTED WITH OXYGEN ● Hydrogen could have reacted with oxygen available from the oxides of Earth's mantle, and could have formed water molecules after our Solar System formed. This water from the mantle could have been later transported to the Earth's surface, forming oceans. [$2 H_2 + O_2 = 2 H_2O$] This theory does not have much supporting evidence and so disregarded.	FALSE!

THE ORIGIN OF THE EARTH'S WATER REVEALED!

🌐 Astronomers, space scientists and academic researchers have known for decades that there is plenty of water in the interstellar medium. There is sufficient scientific research evidence along with journal publications supporting the fact that our planet Earth inherited up to 50% of its water (it is called primordial water) from the interstellar medium even before before our Solar System was created some 6 billion years ago, and the remaining water was believed and proved to have obtained from the bombardment of asteroids (meteorites/ carbonaceous chondrites) during and after the early stages of the formation of our planet Earth in our Solar System.

🌐 The water samples taken from our Earth's deep mantle (rocks found in 1985 from the Baffin Island, Nunavut Territory, Canada) were analysed and proved to contain primordial water formed in the interstellar medium. This discovery has given the strong supporting evidence that the water we drink today is at least 4.54 billion years old, older than our Solar System.

How Did the Water Get Into The Interstellar Medium?

🌐 Nearly 380,000 years after the Big Bang, the primary element "hydrogen" was first created, and thereafter it was abundantly available throughout our Universe. Nearly 400 million years after the Big Bang, stars formation commenced using hydrogen as the burning fuel. The massive pressure build-up of the fiery inferno within the stars was so great that hydrogen atoms fused together to form heavier element helium, and helium atoms in turn fused together to form much heavier elements such as lithium, beryllium, carbon, nitrogen, oxygen, and others in a process known as "**stellar nucleosynthesis**." The early stars were massive and short-lived. When the massive stars finished burning their hydrogen or helium fuel, they eventually extinguished, collapsed as they could not withstand their own gravitational force, and exploded into supernovae while manufacturing, dumping and scattering all kinds of heavier elements such as "carbon, nitrogen, oxygen, phosphorus and sulfur and many other elements" across the interstellar medium of our Milky Way Galaxy, and perhaps across the other galaxies our Universe.

🌐 More than 6 billion years ago, even before our Solar System and our Earth were created, during the supernova explosions in our Milky Way Galaxy, those newly formed heavier elements, including the very important oxygen, commingled together and formed all kinds of newer elements that we see in our periodic table today (there are 117 heavier elements).
Space scientists discovered that during the time when newer elements were being formed, the abundantly available hydrogen and oxygen commingled together in the star-forming clouds under the appropriate climate conditions, and formed ice-cold water molecules by the chemical reaction ($2 H_2 + O_2 = 2 H_2O$). Those ice-cold water molecules then entered into the space dust (also known as stardust) and interstellar gas in the interstellar medium, from a gigantic cloud of which our Solar System (our Sun, our planet Earth & 7 other planets) was created 6 billion years ago. The formation of our Solar System completed 4.54 billion years ago. And that is how our planet Earth inherited liquid water even before it was born. Our planet Earth was thus born with water.
🌐 **The intriguing idea** is that the ices from the interstellar medium were incorporated with a lot of organic material in them, which could have helped kick-start the life on our planet Earth.

CONCLUSION: The Water We Drink Today Is At Least 4.54 Billion Years Old, Older Than Our Planet Earth, Older Than Our Sun, and Older Than Our Solar System! Our planet Earth inherited up to 50% of its water from the interstellar medium even before it was born, and the remaining water came to our planet Earth by the bombardment of Asteroids (not Comets) during and after the early stages of our Solar System formation.
Please refer to APPENDIX-A (Chapter 20) for the detailed scientific studies and complete evidence, including journal publications, on water formation on our planet Earth.

DRINKING WATER STATISTICS AT A GLANCE [77]

Please take a hard look at the following jaw-dropping statistics, posted by the World Health Organization (WHO) in 2018, and avoid becoming another statistic:

- Globally, at least 2 billion people use a drinking water source contaminated with faeces.
- Contaminated water can transmit water-borne diseases such as diarrhea, cholera, malaria, dysentery, typhoid, polio and other illnesses.
- Toxic chemicals arsenic, lead, chromium, beryllium or nickel could cause kidney damage, cancer, birth defects, and other illnesses if you drink contaminated tap water.
- Contaminated drinking water is estimated to cause 502,000 diarrhea deaths each year.
- By the year 2025, half of the world's population will be living in water stressed areas.
- In low and middle-income countries, 38% of health care facilities lack any water source, 19% do not have improved sanitation, and 35% lack water and soap for hand washing.
- It is being reported on the TV channels and in newspapers in USA and in many other countries that many children in schools are being exposed to lead-poison after drinking contaminated tap water in the campuses of schools. This is an alarming news to us because many schools fail to exercise appropriate caution in providing clean and purified water to children.

LIVE LIKE AN ADVANCED HUMAN BEING (RECOMMENDATIONS by Dr. RK)

- Please do not drink tap water, well water, or bottled water of any kind directly without knowing how pure it is. Please always drink purified water (RO water, distilled water, or other).

- Learn how to monitor water pH by using pH testing drops, and urine pH by using pH paper.
- Also learn how to monitor TDS level of water by using a TDS meter. The TDS level of purified water (RO water) should be under 5 ppm. The TDS level of distilled water should be zero.
- Also learn how to test for chlorine and fluoride in your drinking water using test strips every now and then. The allowable chlorine level in drinking water is up to 5 ppm or mg/L.
The allowable fluoride level in drinking water is 1.5 for children and 2.4 ppm or mg/L for adults.

- World Health Organization (WHO) reported that drinking water with no minerals is potentially harmful to human health. So learn how to remineralize the purified water by adding Himalayan pink salt, Celtic sea salt, or ConcenTrace mineral drops to purified water. Learn how to remineralize the purified water up to a TDS (Total Dissolved Solids) level of 200 ppm.
- Or purchase a reliable pitcher that purifies tap water, adds minerals, and raises pH. Make sure that the pitcher is working perfectly by testing the water with a TDS meter and a pH meter.
- Get your drinking water tested by a certified laboratory in your area frequently, and make sure that the water you drink is one hundred percent free of contaminants.
- Consume one whole lemon a day including the pulp to neutralize your body's urine. Learn how to raise the pH of purified water by adding a tiny bit of baking soda or by adding ConcenTrace mineral drops. Make sure that the pH of your drinking water is 7, or between 7 and 7.25. Please do not drink the water that is acidic (If the water pH is below 7, that is acidic). Learn how to neutralize or slightly alkalize the purified water before drinking.
- There were many reported health benefits of alkaline ionized water, Kangen water, hydrogen water, and alkaline RO water. Learn how to make your own alkaline water, and start drinking alkaline water periodically (not every day), and get you blood pH tested routinely. Normal blood pH should be between 7.35 and 7.45. By trial and error, find out how much alkaline water would suit your body and help feel healthy. Adjust your drinking water pH until it suits your body.

- Drinking Water Guide teaches you everything you need on how to remineralize and alkalize the purified water at the comfort of your home without purchasing expensive purification systems.
- The RECOMMENDATIONS provided by the author at the end of each chapter would guide you on what exactly you need to do to protect your health.
- You are about to discover very many extremely useful drinking water strategies in this book, so please proceed to the next chapter and the following chapters.

REFERENCES

AMAZING FACTS ABOUT OUR UNIVERSE, OUR STARS, OUR MILKY WAY GALAXY, OUR SOLAR SYSTEM, OUR SUN & OUR EARTH!

AGE OF OUR UNIVERSE
1. How Old is the Universe? by NASA (The National Aeronautics and Space Administration), NASA posted that we can estimate the age of the universe to be about 13.77 ± 0.059 billion years! Posted on Dec 21, 2012.
https://wmap.gsfc.nasa.gov/universe/uni_age.html

2. Age of the Universe, Wilkinson Microwave Anisotropy Probe, From Wikipedia, the free encyclopedia, Last edited Feb 21, 2019. NASA's Wilkinson Microwave Anisotropy Probe (WMAP) estimated in 2012 the age of the universe to be 13.772 billion years, with an uncertainty of plus or minus 59 million years. The current measurement of the age of the universe is approximately 13.8 billion years.
https://en.wikipedia.org/wiki/Age_of_the_universe
https://en.wikipedia.org/wiki/Wilkinson_Microwave_Anisotropy_Probe

3. How Old Is The Universe?, Frequently Asked Questions by Hubblesite.org.
The universe is approximately 13.8 billion years old.
https://hubblesite.org/quick-facts/science-quick-facts
https://hubblesite.org/quick-facts/mission-quick-facts

4. How old are galaxies? by NASA Space Place. Our universe is about 13.8 billion years old, and our own Milky Way galaxy is approximately 13.6 billion years old. Article last updated on, Jan 24, 2019, Posted on March 12, 2019, Last updated on Sept 16, 2020.
https://spaceplace.nasa.gov/galaxies-age/en/

5. How Old is the Universe? "In 2012, WMAP estimated the age of the universe to be 13.772 billion years, with an uncertainty of 59 million years" by Nola Taylor Redd, Posted on June 08, 2017, Science & Astronomy, Space.com.
https://www.space.com/24054-how-old-is-the-universe.html

HOW MANY STARS ARE THERE IN OUR UNIVERSE?
6. How many stars are there in the Universe? by European Space Agency. There are 10^{11} to 10^{12} stars in our Galaxy, and there are perhaps something like 10^{11} or 10^{12} galaxies. Simple calculation gives you 10^{22} to 10^{24} stars in the Universe.
https://www.esa.int/Our_Activities/Space_Science/Herschel/How_many_stars_are_there_in_the_Universe
https://www.esa.int/Science_Exploration/Space_Science/Herschel/How_many_stars_are_there_in_the_Universe

7. How many Stars in the Universe? by Fraser Cain, Posted on January 03, 2013.
If you multiply the number of stars in our galaxy by the number of galaxies in the Universe, you get approximately 10^{24} stars (That's a 1 followed by twenty-four zeros).
https://www.universetoday.com/102630/how-many-stars-are-there-in-the-universe/

HOW MANY GALAXIES ARE THERE IN OUR UNIVERSE?
8. Galaxy, From Wikipedia, the free encyclopedia, Number of galaxies in the observable universe has been changed from a previous estimate of 200 billion (2×10^{11}) to a suggested current estimate of 2 trillion (2×10^{12}) or more, Posted on March 7, 2017. https://en.wikipedia.org/wiki/Galaxy

9. Hubble Reveals "Observable Universe Contains 10 Times More Galaxies Than Previously Thought," by Editor Karl Hille, Nasa.gov, Posted on Oct 13, 2016, Updated on Aug 6, 2017. https://www.nasa.gov/feature/goddard/2016/hubble-reveals-observable-universe-contains-10-times-more-galaxies-than-previously-thought

10. This Is How We Know There Are Two Trillion Galaxies In The Universe by Ethan Siegel, PhD, Senior Contributor, Science, Posted on Forbes.com. https://www.forbes.com/sites/startswithabang/2018/10/18/this-is-how-we-know-there-are-two-trillion-galaxies-in-the-universe/#79bb52055a67

HOW OLD IS OUR MILKY WAY GALAXY?

11. How old are galaxies? "Milky Way galaxy is approximately 13.6 billion years old." Posted by NASA Space Place, Article last updated on March 12, 2019. https://spaceplace.nasa.gov/galaxies-age/en/

12. Milky Way Facts by The Planets. The oldest star in the Galaxy is HD 140283, also known as the "Methuselah Star," and it is at least 13.6 billion years old. https://theplanets.org/milky-way/

13. Milky Way's Age Narrowed Down (The study puts its age at 13.6 billion years, give or take 800 million years) by Robert Roy Britt, Space.com, Posted on August 17, 2004. https://www.space.com/263-milky-age-narrowed.html

HOW MANY SOLAR SYSTEMS ARE IN OUR MILKY WAY GALAXY?

14. How Many Stars in the Milky Way? by Maggie Masetti, Posted on July 22, 2015. There are 100 billion stars in the Milky Way on the low-end and 400 billion on the high end. https://asd.gsfc.nasa.gov/blueshift/index.php/2015/07/22/how-many-stars-in-the-milky-way/

15. Astronomy Course "Exploring the Universe" Being Offered at eDynamic Learning by Edgenuity.com. Our Sun is just one of approximately 500 billion stars in our galaxy, meaning that there could possibly be up to 500 billion solar systems. https://www.edgenuity.com/Syllabi/edynamics/EDL028-Syllabus_Astronomy.pdf

16. ASTRONOMY Course Being Offered at the National University Virtual High School, Chula Vista, CA 91910-5200, USA, Posted in April 2016. Our Sun is just one of approximately 500 billion stars in our galaxy, meaning that there could possibly be up to 500 billion solar systems. https://www.nuvhs.org/assets/resources/courseResources/Syllabus_Astronomy1.pdf

17. Milky Way, From Wikipedia, the free encyclopedia, March 9, 2019. Milky Way Galaxy is estimated to contain 100–400 billion stars and as many as 100-400 billion planets. https://en.wikipedia.org/wiki/Milky_Way

18. How Many Stars Are in the Milky Way? by Elizabeth Howell, Space.com, Posted on March 30, 2018. Talks about counting stars by determining the galaxy's mass, dark energy, etc. The estimate of the total stars in our Milky Way Galaxy at 100 billion (based on solar mass). https://www.space.com/25959-how-many-stars-are-in-the-milky-way.html

19. The Milky Way Galaxy, Imagine the Universe by NASA.gov, Goddard Space Flight Center. Milky Way is made up of approximately 100 billion stars (This information is outdated). It takes 250 million years for our Sun and our entire solar system to go all the way around the center of our Milky Way Galaxy. https://imagine.gsfc.nasa.gov/science/objects/milkyway1.html

20. How many solar systems are in our galaxy? Sun is one of about 200 billion stars (or perhaps more) just in the Milky Way galaxy alone, Posted by Spacespace of Nasa.
https://spaceplace.nasa.gov/review/dr-marc-space/solar-systems-in-galaxy.html

21. The Reference # 21 is not assigned and not being used.

FORMATION OF OUR UNIVERSE: BIG BANG THEORY

22. Discovery of the Cosmic Microwave Background (CMB), Our Universe, WMAP's Universe by NASA.gov, Posted and Updated on Sept 05, 2016.
https://wmap.gsfc.nasa.gov/universe/bb_tests_cmb.html

23. The Universe: Big Bang to Now in 10 Easy Steps by Denise Chow, Science & Astronomy, Posted on October 19, 2011. https://www.space.com/13320-big-bang-universe-10-steps-explainer.html

24. Origin of Universe and Big Bang Theory, Published on Slideshare by Salim Lakade, Student at Latthe Polytechnic, Sangli, Maharashtra State, India, Published on Sep 8, 2017.
https://www.slideshare.net/salimlakade/origin-of-universe-big-bang-theory

25. Step by Step of The Big Bang Theory by jonval21, Steemit Social Media Network.
https://steemit.com/universe/@jonval21/step-by-step-of-the-big-bang-theory

26. The SIX Things you may not know about the afterglow of the Big Bang by Physics.org.
http://www.physics.org/featuredetail.asp?id=45

27. Our Expanding Universe: Age, History & Other Facts by Charles Q. Choi, Space.com Contributor, Posted on June 17, 2017.
https://www.space.com/52-the-expanding-universe-from-the-big-bang-to-today.html

28. The Early Universe by Las Cumbres Observatory, 6740 Cortona Drive, Suite 102, Goleta, CA 93117, USA, 2019.
https://lco.global/spacebook/early-universe/
https://lco.global/spacebook/cosmology/early-universe/

29. Timeline of the Big Bang by The Physics of the Universe, 2019.
https://www.physicsoftheuniverse.com/topics_bigbang_timeline.html

PRIMORDIAL SOUP CONDITION RECREATED BY CERN, SWITZERLAND

30. Big Bang 'soup recipe' confirmed by Rolf Haugaard Nielse, Posted on June 13, 2003.
https://www.newscientist.com/article/dn3821-big-bang-soup-recipe-confirmed/

31. Scientists at CERN Catch a Glimpse of the Universe's Primordial Soup by Todd Jaquith, Posted on Feb 10, 2016.
https://futurism.com/scientists-at-cern-catch-a-glimpse-of-the-universes-primordial-soup

32. LHC (Large Hadron Collider) Produces 'Primordial Soup' of The Universe Using Less Particles Than Thought Possible by Bec Crew, Posted on Sep 7, 2015.
https://www.sciencealert.com/lhc-produces-primordial-soup-of-the-universe-using-less-particles-than-thought-possible

33. The Universe's Primordial Soup Flowing at CERN by You Zhou & Jens Jørgen Gaardhøje, Niels Bohr Institute, University of Copenhagen, Denmark, Posted on February 9, 2016.
https://phys.org/news/2016-02-universe-primordial-soup-cern.html
https://www.nbi.ku.dk/english/news/news16/the-universes-primordial-soup-flowing-at-cern/

FORMATION OF OUR UNIVERSE: BIG BANG THEORY (Continued)
34. General Astronomy, The First 3 Minutes by Wikibooks, Posted on Oct 16, 2018.
https://en.wikibooks.org/wiki/General_Astronomy/The_First_Three_Minutes

35. Abundance of the chemical elements, From Wikipedia, the free encyclopedia, Last updated March 27, 2019.
https://en.wikipedia.org/wiki/Abundance_of_the_chemical_elements

36. Chronology of the Universe, From Wikipedia, the free encyclopedia, Updated on March 27, 2019.
https://en.wikipedia.org/wiki/Chronology_of_the_universe
37. First Light & Reionization by NASA.gov.
https://jwst.nasa.gov/firstlight.html

38. YouTube Video, The Big Bang Theory Explained The Simple Way by gphhawkins, Published on Sep 22, 2011.
https://www.youtube.com/watch?v=wt4TmZVS0Do

STELLAR NUCLEOSYNTHESIS
39. Is my body really made up of star stuff? by StarChild Authors (Phil Newman and Others) of NASA.
https://starchild.gsfc.nasa.gov/docs/StarChild/questions/question57.html

40. Stars: Element Factories, Stellar fusion creates most elements in the Universe; "When you look up at night, you are seeing factories called stars" by Kent Fairfield, Lifelong Amateur Astronomer, The Bulletin, Posted on Oct 29, 2014.
https://www.bendbulletin.com/outdoors/2523761-151/stars-element-factories

41. Stellar Nuceosynthesis, How elements from helium and hydrogen are created by Andrew Zimmerman Jones, Updated on December 07, 2018.
https://www.thoughtco.com/stellar-nucleosynthesis-2699311

42. NASA Finds a "Weird" Kind of Life on Earth. Life requires the six elements CHNOPS (carbon, hydrogen, nitrogen, oxygen, phosphorus and sulfur), Posted by Nancy Atkinson, Universe Today, Space and Astronomy News, December 2, 2010.
http://www.universetoday.com/81106/nasa-finds-a-weird-kind-of-life-on-earth/

43. What are the Ingredients of Life? Posted by Natalie Wolchover, February 02, 2011.
All organisms are built from the same six essential elemental ingredients: carbon, hydrogen, nitrogen, oxygen, phosphorus and sulfur (CHNOPS).
https://www.livescience.com/32983-what-are-ingredients-life.html#~:text=Nonetheless%2C%20all%20organisms%20are%20built,Why%20those%20elements%3F

44. Dr. Carl Sagan, "Cosmos," Paperback, Ann Druyan (Introduction), Neil deGrasse Tyson (Foreword), ISBN number 978-0345539434, Amazon.com, December 10, 2013.

45. Composition of the human body, From Wikipedia, the free encyclopedia.
https://en.wikipedia.org/wiki/Composition_of_the_human_body#~:text=Almost%2099%25%20of%20the%20mass,11%20are%20necessary%20for%20life

FORMATION OF OUR MILKY WAY GALAXY

46. What is a galaxy (galaxy pictures posted)? by Space Place of Nasa.gov.
https://spaceplace.nasa.gov/galaxy/en/

47. Why Do We Call Our Galaxy the Milky Way? by Deanna Kerley, Posted on November 13, 2013.
http://mentalfloss.com/article/53589/why-do-we-call-our-galaxy-milky-way

48. How Did the Milky Way Get Its Name? by Mindy Weisberger, Senior Writer, Posted on November 7, 2016.
https://www.livescience.com/56756-milky-way-name-origin.html

References from 49 to 54 are not assigned and not being used.

FORMATION OF OUR SOLAR SYSTEM

55. Mysteries of the Universe (The picture of a nebula posted) by Nasa.gov. Pillars of Creation, Eagle Nebula, a cloud of gas and dust created by an exploding star from which new stars and planets are forming.
https://www.nasa.gov/specials/60counting/universe.html
https://www.nasa.gov/image-feature/the-pillars-of-creation
https://www.nasa.gov/image-feature/eagle-nebula-s-pillars-of-creation-in-infrared

56. How to build a solar system (The picture of a nebula posted) by Karla Panchuk, Department of Geological Sciences, University of Saskatchewan, Canada.
https://opentextbc.ca/geology/chapter/22-3-how-to-build-a-solar-system/

FORMATION OF OUR PLANET EARTH

57. How Planets Are Born, Story by Alison Takemura, Posted on June 16, 2016.
https://nasaviz.gsfc.nasa.gov/12278

58. Our Sun Came Late to the Milky Way's Star-Birth Party by Donna Weaver, Editor: Lynn Jenner, Space Telescope Science Institute, Baltimore, Maryland, Posted & Updated on Aug. 6, 2017.
https://www.nasa.gov/content/goddard/our-sun-came-late-to-the-milky-way-s-star-birth-party

59. Did a Supernova Give Birth to Our Solar System? by Charles Q. Choi, Space.com Contributor, Posted on December 28, 2016.
https://www.space.com/35151-supernova-trigger-solar-system-formation.html

60. Solar System Formation, Windows to the Universe, Brought to you by the National Earth Science Teachers Association, 2012.
https://www.windows2Universe.org/our_solar_system/formation.html

THE SIZE OF OUR SUN & LIFESPAN OF OUR SUN

61. How large is the Sun compared to Earth? Posted by Cool Cosmos.
https://coolcosmos.ipac.caltech.edu/ask/5-How-large-is-the-Sun-compared-to-Earth-

61b. How Hot Is the Sun? by Tim Sharp, Reference Editor, Posted on October 18, 2017.
The sun is about 93 million miles (149.5 million km) from Earth.
https://www.space.com/17137-how-hot-is-the-sun.html
61c. How do scientists know the distance between the planets? by the Spaceplace of NASA.
The Sun is about 93 million miles from Earth.
https://spaceplace.nasa.gov/review/dr-marc-solar-system/planet-distances.html

62. How old is the Sun?, NASA Space Place, Posted on March 12, 2019. Our Sun is 4.54 billion years old. Stars like our Sun burn for about 9 or 10 billion years. So our Sun is about halfway through its life.
https://spaceplace.nasa.gov/sun-age/en/

FORMATION OF OUR MOON
63. YouTube Title: Whole Story from the Big Bang to the Present Day - Full Documentary (History of the World in 2 Hours) by Perfect Toys, Published on Apr 24, 2016. Narrators: Alex Filippenko (Astrophysicist), Peter Ward (Paleontologist), Clifford V. Johnson (Physicist, University of Southern California), and others.
https://www.youtube.com/watch?v=_ITHx8SKD5g   (This vodeo is unavailable now!)

64. History of the World in 2 Hours by Alex Filippenko (Astrophysicist), Peter Ward (Paleontologist), and others, DVD, ASIN: B006ENHGLS, Available on Amazon.com.

AGE OF OUR PLANET EARTH BY RADIOMATRIC DATING
65. The Earth is 18 Galactic Years Old, Astronomy, Earth Facts, Posted on January 16, 2018. The age of the Earth is approximately 4.54 billion years.
https://ourplnt.com/Earth-18-galactic-years-old/

66. Dear Science: How do we know how old the Earth is? by Sarah Kaplan March 6, 2017. Researchers used uranium-lead techniques to date the meteorite back 4.54 billion years, give or take about 70 million — the best age for our planet so far, according to the U.S. Geological Survey.
https://www.washingtonpost.com/news/speaking-of-science/wp/2017/03/06/dear-science-how-do-we-know-how-old-the-earth-is/?noredirect=on&utm_term=.c0d5c099c3a5

67. How Old Is Earth? by Nola Taylor Redd, Science & Astronomy, Space.com, February 07, 2019.
https://www.space.com/24854-how-old-is-earth.html

68. Age of the Earth – Timeline by Science Learning Hub, Updated on April 22, 2014. Chronological order of scientific discoveries of the measurement of the age of the Earth.
https://www.sciencelearn.org.nz/resources/1553-age-of-the-earth-timeline

69. How old is the Earth?, Posted by NASA.gov. Earth's age: About 4.5 billion years based on radioactive dating using uranium and thorium isotopes.
https://image.gsfc.nasa.gov/poetry/ask/a10597.html

70. Age of the Earth, From Wikipedia, the free encyclopedia, Last edited on March 11, 2019. The age of the Earth is 4.54 ± 0.05 billion years (4.54 × 109 years ± 1%)
https://en.wikipedia.org/wiki/Age_of_the_Earth

71. How is Earth's Age Calculated? by Jeanna Bryner, Live Science Managing Editor, Posted on November 29, 2012.
https://www.livescience.com/32321-how-is-earths-age-calculated.html

ABOUT OUR PLANET EARTH

72. Space and Astronomy News, Universe Today, Posted on Feb 10, 2017. Our planet Earth has a surface area of approximately 510 million square kilometers or 196.9 million square miles. https://www.universetoday.com/25756/surface-area-of-the-earth/

73. Our Sun by the Numbers, Solar System Exploration by NASA.gov. Our planet Earth has a surface area of approximately 510 million square kilometers or 196.9 million square miles. https://solarsystem.nasa.gov/solar-system/sun/by-the-numbers/

74. World population projected to reach 9.8 billion in 2050, and 11.2 billion in 2100, by United Nations, Dept of Economics and Social Affairs, Posted in 2017. https://www.un.org/development/desa/en/news/population/world-population-prospects-2017.html

75. How much water is there on, in, and above the Earth? by US Geological Survey (USGS) Water Science School, Posted on Dec 2, 2016. https://water.usgs.gov/edu/earthhowmuch.html

WATER FORMATION ON OUR PLANET EARTH

76. Oceans Worlds, Water in the Solar System and Beyond by NASA. According to NASA's report, there are more than 326 million trillion gallons of liquid water on our Earth. https://www.nasa.gov/specials/ocean-worlds/

77. Drinking Water Statistics by World Health Organization (WHO), Posted on Feb 07, 2018. http://www.who.int/news-room/fact-sheets/detail/drinking-water http://www.who.int/en/news-room/fact-sheets/detail/drinking-water

APPENDIX-A
CHAPTER 20: THE ORIGIN OF THE EARTH'S WATER
WATER FORMATION ON OUR PLANET EARTH
(CONTINUATION OF CHAPTER 1)

TABLE OF CONTENTS

<u>Did you know?</u>
The oxygen we breathe today was originally created in the Stars
even before our Solar System was created!
The water we drink today was originally created in the stars-forming clouds
even before our Solar System was created!
When you look up at night, you are seeing factories called Stars!

FORMATION OF OUR UNIVERSE: SUMMARY

● Our Universe is about 13.8 billion years old. The NASA's Wilkinson Microwave Anisotropy Probe (WMAP) mission precisely determined the age of our Universe.

● <u>Our Universe was born 13.8 billion years ago with the Big Bang</u> as an unbelievably and unimaginably hot and dense point of singularity, which was at infinite temperature and infinite density. When our Universe was just 10^{-34} of a second young — that is, when it was a hundredth of a billionth of a trillionth of a trillionth of a second young — it underwent an incredible burst of expansion known as inflation, in which period the space itself expanded like a magical balloon faster than the speed of light, and doubled its size at least 90 consecutive times. At that very beginning stage of formation, our Universe existed in the form of quark-gluon plasma, also called the primordial soup. No stable atoms were created yet.

● <u>Nearly one second after the Big Bang</u>, the temperature of our Universe dropped to 1 billion degrees or 10^9 degrees Kelvin, and as a result, the most fundamental particles such as quarks, electrons, photons and neutrinos just formed, but not yet bound together.
<u>Nearly 3 minutes after the Big Bang</u>, our Universe underwent a cooling process in which the quarks coalesced and bound into hadrons such as protons and neutrons. It was called hadrons era. The protons and neutrons in turn combined to form nuclei of light elements such as hydrogen and helium (no neutral atoms were created yet). This is one of the most important events of the history of the Big Bang because our visible Universe today is composed of 90% hydrogen, 8% helium, and 2% everything else.

● <u>Nearly 380,000 years after the Big Bang, the primary element "hydrogen" was created, and thereafter hydrogen was abundantly available throughput our Universe. The nuclei of the light elements such as hydrogen, helium, lithium and beryllium attracted electrons, and formed neutral atoms (stable atoms formed) in a process known as "stellar nucleosynthesis"</u>. This is one of the most important events of the history of the Big Bang because our visible Universe today is composed of 90% hydrogen, 8% helium, and 2% everything else.

● Our Universe kept expanding unstoppably and unimaginably without boundaries, and the temperature kept dropping exponentially. Our Universe then entered into an era of dark ages for 100s of millions of years because there were no stars.

● <u>Nearly 400 million years after the Big Bang</u>, stars formation commenced, as clumps of gas collapsed enough under gravity while spinning and swirling took place to form the very first bright light, which became a star, thereby creating the first star, and followed by more and more stars, and eventually millions of stars along with the orbiting planets.

● The early stars were massive and made up of very simple and light gaseous elements (hydrogen and helium) and so they had very short lifespans of only millions of years. But the fiery inferno and nuclear fusion in the cores of these early stars slowly created all kinds of heavier elements (there are 117 heavier elements in our periodic table), including the most important Carbon, Nitrogen, Oxygen, Phosphorus and Sulfur. When a large star died, it would become a part of a new star in the supernova explosion. In the beginning, these stars were created in small groups and attracted other stars. These stars were grouped in both regular and irregular shapes. Then the different shapes merged to form the first galaxies. Then as more and more galaxies formed, they became grouped in galaxy clusters, and then these clusters were contained in super clusters.

● Likewise, our Universe has been creating millions of stars along with orbiting planets and galaxies, and then billions of stars along with orbiting planets and galaxies, and then even trillions of stars along with orbiting planets and galaxies that are visible today!

FORMATION OF OUR SOLAR SYSTEM, OUR SUN, AND OUR PLANET EARTH
Did You Know Stars Manufacture Planets Like Factories Do?

◉ Our Solar System began its formation some 6 billion years ago. A gigantic interstellar cloud known as solar nebula of space dust and gas that was squeezed by a supernova explosion gave birth to our Solar System. The solid particles glued together along with the gas, and the resulting mass by spinning and swirling made circular orbits. The gentle collisions allowed the solid flakes to stick together and to make larger particles which, in turn, attracted more solid particles. This process of spinning and swirling, and accretion of space dust and gas continued for 100s of millions of years, or even billions of years, until the larger solid balls of accretion formed, and gave birth to 8 planets, including our planet Earth. The formation of our Sun along with the orbiting 8 planets completed 4.54 billion years ago.

◉ Near the center of the burning Sun where only rocky material could stand the great heat, the four terrestrial or inner planets "**Mercury, Venus, Earth and Mars**" formed. And away from the centre of the burning Sun or farther to the burning Sun, icy and gassy matter settled in the outer regions of the disk, where the other four giant or jovian outer planets "**Jupiter, Saturn, Uranus and Neptune**" formed.

◉ Our scientists determined the age of our planet Earth as 4.54 billion years by radiometric dating, which is the most accurate and reliable method to date old rocks. Our Solar System (and all the items in it) is therefore 4.54 billion years old.

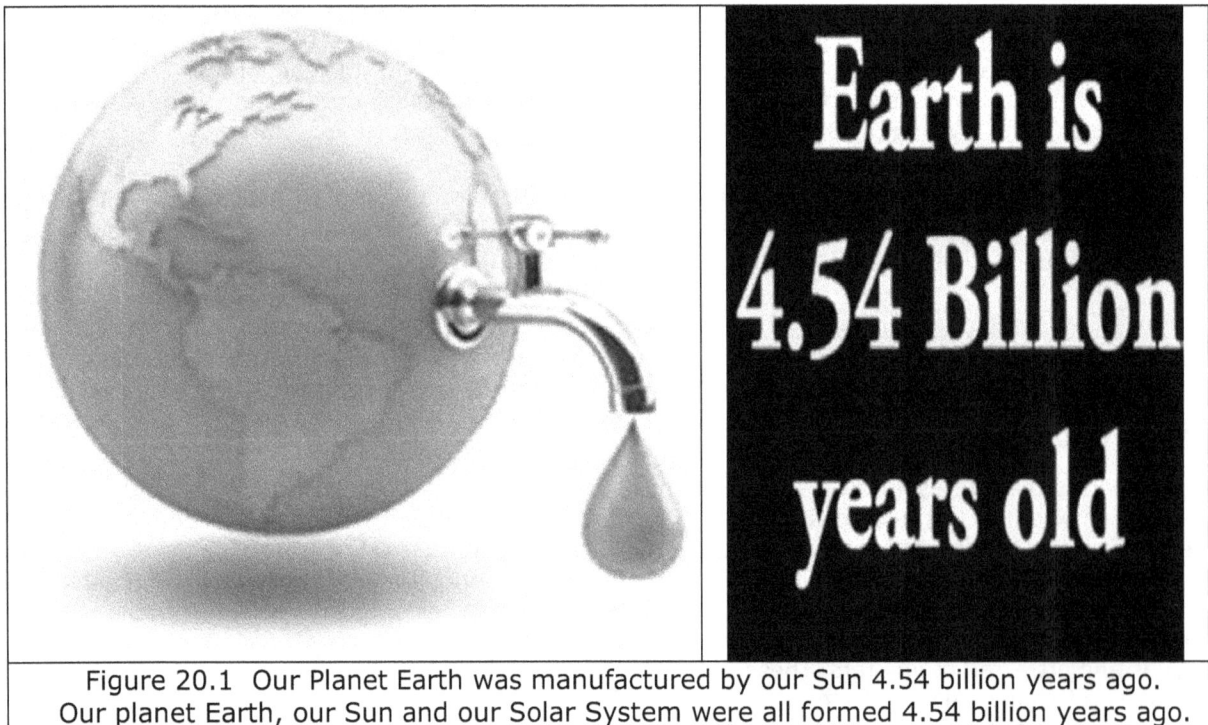

Earth is 4.54 Billion years old

Figure 20.1 Our Planet Earth was manufactured by our Sun 4.54 billion years ago.
Our planet Earth, our Sun and our Solar System were all formed 4.54 billion years ago.

WATER FORMATION ON OUR PLANET EARTH

Water is the principal ingredient necessary for the life formation. Without water, we wouldn't have been be here on the planet Earth!

How Much Water The Earth Had?: About 71% of our Earth's surface is covered by water, cycling through oceans, rivers and lakes, and recycling through clouds. About 60% of our bodied are made up of water. There are more than 326 million trillion gallons of water on Earth. Earth's oceans contain about 96.5 percent of all the planet's water. Less than 3 percent of all water on Earth is freshwater that is usable for drinkable. More than two-thirds of Earth's freshwater is locked up in ice caps and glaciers. Earth isn't the only ocean world in our Solar System. Scientists believe that water on other worlds exists in diverse forms on moons, dwarf planets, comets, asteroids, and meteorites. Frozen ice, water vapor in the atmosphere, and oceans on the other worlds offer clues in the quest to discover life beyond our home planet. [80]

Water is Everywhere: Astronomers believe that Jupiter's moons "Europa and Callisto," Saturn's tiny moon "Enceladus" and the red planet "Mars" may contain liquid water and even the oceans, beneath the surface of the frozen ice crust. Most of the water in other places of our galaxy is thought to be in the form of frozen ice or water vapor. Liquid water similar to the one in our Earth is hard to find. [81]

Water Formation in our Universe: Astronomers say that water is everywhere in our Milky Way Galaxy. Hydrogen is the first abundant element found in our Universe and in our galaxy. About 75% of all atoms in our galaxy are hydrogen atoms. Helium is the second most abundant element, and oxygen is the third most abundant element. Water [H_2O] is made from two hydrogen atoms and one oxygen atom. Water forms anywhere in our Milky Way Galaxy and in our Universe as long as the appropriate conditions prevail:

(i) Both hydrogen and oxygen must abundantly be available under appropriate climate conditions (temperatures below -223 °C or 50 °K may be necessary in most cases), and
(ii) the ionization of hydrogen molecules should readily be possible in order to take place the chemical reaction.[82]

Hydrogen was first created nearly 380,000 years after the Big Bang when our Universe was born. But oxygen was not available in our Universe until and after some 400 million years when the first stars were born. During the first stars formation and beyond, both hydrogen and oxygen were abundantly available throughout our Universe and more specifically in our Milky Way Galaxy. Oxygen is made in stars when the primitive elements such as hydrogen, helium and lithium were fused to form many other heavier elements, and dispersed out into our Universe in events such as supernova explosions. The two elements "hydrogen and oxygen" react in star-forming clouds and form large amounts of water [$2 H_2 + O_2 = 2 H_2O$]. The molecules of water leave the clouds of dust and gas, and end up in many different places – planets, comets, asteroids, and meteorites.

WATER FORMATION ON OUR PLANET EARTH (5 THEORIES)? [80-166]

The puzzling question on everyone's mind is: **"How did the Earth possess that much water (more than 326 million trillion gallons)?"** Astronomers, space researchers, scientists and very many academic researchers have been struggling to find out the truth through out the human history, but were unable to come up with a definitive answer thus far. However all those scientific research findings can be summarized into the following 5 theories. These 5 theories are discussed in detail along with journal publications in Chapter 20.

THEORIES OF WATER FORMATION ON OUR EARTH	CONCLUSION
1. COMETS COULD HAVE BROUGHT WATER TO EARTH • Our Solar System (Our Sun, Our Earth and other 7 Planets) began its formation 6 billion years ago, and completed its formation 4.54 billion years ago. Our ancestors believed that ice-bearing comets probably bombarded our Earth 4 to 3.8 billion years ago, and brought water to Earth. This theory is now believed to be wrong because (D/H Ratio) of the water from comets is much higher than that of ocean water. Our ancestors' belief that comets brought water to our planet Earth was however proved by our most recent scientists to be a myth.	MYTH!
2. ASTEROIDS (METEORITES /CARBONACEOUS CHONDRITES) COULD HAVE BROUGHT WATER TO EARTH • Water-rich asteroids (meteorites / carbonaceous chondrites) impacted the infant Earth about 4 to 3.8 billion years ago, distributing water across the planet by brute force. As a result, our oceans formed. This theory is more accurate because D/H Ratio of the water from asteroids matched well with that of ocean water. Research proved that our planet Earth attained up to 50% of its water from the asteroids during the early stages after the formation of our Solar System.	TRUE!
3. EARTH INHERITED ITS WATER FROM THE INTERSTELLAR MEDIUM • Water is known to form in the clouds of gas and dust of the interstellar medium (ISM). Our Solar System was created 6 billion years ago from a gigantic cloud of interstellar gas and stardust. That cloud collapsed and formed a solar nebula—a spinning, swirling disk of material under gravity. Scientists found that the primordial water of the interstellar medium survived within the particles of the stardust, and carried forward all the way until and after the formation our Earth. Researchers concluded, from an extensive experimental study and mathematical modelling, that our planet Earth inherited up to 50% of its water from the interstellar medium even before our Solar System was created. Our Solar System completed its formation 4.54 billion years ago. However the water we drink today is at least 4.54 billion years old.	TRUE!
4. EARTH'S DEEP MANTLE HAS THE PRIMORDIAL WATER FROM THE INTERSTELLAR MEDIUM • The researchers collected samples of primitive rocks from the Baffin Island, Nunavut Territory, Canada back in 1985. Water analysis revealed that these rocks have lower amount of deuterium, and lower D/H Ratio, indicating that the Earth's deep mantle attained the primordial water from the interstellar medium. Which means the water we drink today is at least 4.54 billion years old.	TRUE!
5. THICK HYDROGEN LAYER COULD HAVE REACTED WITH OXYGEN • Hydrogen could have reacted with oxygen available from the oxides of Earth's mantle, and could have formed water molecules after our Solar System formed. This water from the mantle could have been later transported to the Earth's surface, forming oceans. [$2 H_2 + O_2 = 2 H_2O$] This theory does not have much supporting evidence and so disregarded.	FALSE!

All the above-mentioned theories are discussed in the following pages. Scientists have developed methods to either credit or discredit a water-formation theory by analysing and monitoring the amount of "deuterium" present in water and by comparing the (D/H Ratio) in any given sample with that of ocean water. So in order to understand "The Origin of the Earth's Water," you should at first understand what the Deuterium is all about.

WHAT IS DEUTERIUM?

The deuterium, also called heavy hydrogen, is an isotope of hydrogen. In Greek language, deutero means "second." The term Deuterium was used to denote the two particles composing the nucleus. Deuterium was first discovered and named in 1931 by Harold Urey (An American Physical Chemist). When the neutron was discovered in 1932, this made the nuclear structure of deuterium obvious, and Harold Urey won the Nobel Prize in 1934. Soon after deuterium's discovery, Harold Urey and others produced samples of heavy water in which the deuterium content had been highly concentrated. [83]

Isotopes are atoms that have the same number of protons and electrons but different numbers of neutrons and therefore have different atomic masses and physical properties.

Hydrogen has more than 3 isotopes: protium (the most common form of hydrogen), deuterium, tritium, and others.

a. Protium (H_1^1): It has 1 proton, 1 electron and 0 neutron (no neutrons).
b. Deuterium (H_1^2): It has 1 proton, 1 electron and 1 neutron.
c. Tritium (H_1^3): It has 1 proton, 1 electron and 2 neutrons.

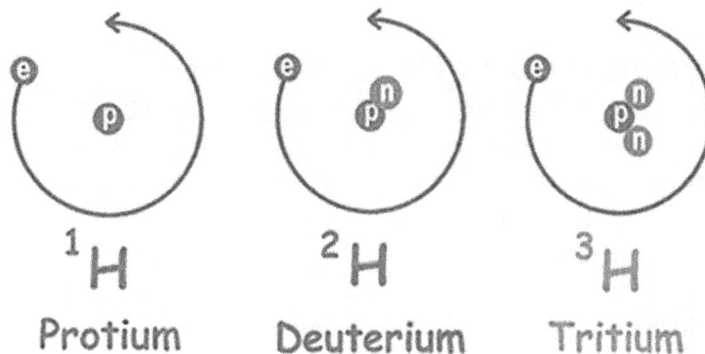

^1H ^2H ^3H
Protium   Deuterium   Tritium

Figure 20.2 Picture showing three isotopes of hydrogen.

The most common form of hydrogen is protium, which refers to the primary isotope of the element hydrogen. When anyone is talking about hydrogen, that refers to protium. Deuterium is the secondary isotope of hydrogen, available in our Universe in only trace amounts.

Elemental Hydrogen exists as a diatomic molecule consisting of two individual Hydrogen atoms bound to one another chemically. The chemical formula is H2. The atom H does not exist as a lone H, at least not naturally. But rather naturally occurring H is H_2.

Normal Water Vs Heavy Water [84]

a. Two hydrogen atoms and one oxygen atom makes a water molecule; Normal water is made up of protium without any presence of deuterium; Heavy water is also water, but it contains a tiny amount of higher isotope called "deuterium."

b. Normal water is composed of dihydrogen oxide molecules (H_2O); Heavy water is composed of deuterium oxide molecules (D_2O)

c. Normal water boils at 100° C; Heavy water boils at 101.4 °C.
   Normal water freezes at 0° C; Heavy water freezes at 3.8° C.
   Ice of normal water floats on the surface of water; Ice of heavy water sinks.

d. The mass of normal water is 18 g/mole; The mass of heavy water is 20 g/mole.

e. Physical properties such as "density, PH value, dynamic viscosity, heat of fusion, heat of vaporization, surface tension and refractive index" of heavy water are relatively higher compared to normal water.

DEUTERIUM FACTS

• The formation of our Universe began with the Big Bang 13.8 billion years ago, and formed atoms, stars, galaxies, and eventually planets. After two minutes of our Universe formation with the Big Bang, deuterium formed by the fusion of protons and neutrons. [85]

• Deuterium is not produced in stars; it is only destroyed in stars. [86]

• Nearly all deuterium found in nature was already produced when the primary element hydrogen was first created 380,000 years after the Big Bang, and the basic or primordial ratio of deuterium-to-hydrogen ((D/H Ratio) is "about 26 atoms of deuterium per million atoms of hydrogen". [83]

• If consumed long term, heavy water (which contains deuterium) can cause harmful side effects to your health as it destroys the metabolism process, and so daily consumption of heavy water is not recommended.

DEUTERIUM-TO-HYDROGEN RATIO (D/H Ratio) [83, 87, 88]

Researchers have been using Deuterium-to-Hydrogen Ratio (D/H Ratio) to identify the origin of water. The basic or primordial (D/H Ratio) at the time of Big Bang is 26 atoms of deuterium per million atoms of hydrogen. The mean (D/H Ratio) for seawater is 156 atoms of deuterium per million atoms of hydrogen.

(D/H Ratio) for the Primordial Water = $26 \times 10^{-6} = 0.26 \times 10^{-4}$
[This ratio is for the water from the Interstellar Medium]

(D/H Ratio) for Seawater = $156 \times 10^{-6} = 1.56 \times 10^{-4}$
[This ratio is for the Earth's Water]

Researchers have compared the (D/H Ratio) of water samples taken from comets, asteroids (meteorites / carbonaceous chondrites), and concluded that the (D/H Ratio) of asteroids matched well with that of seawater, but did not match with that of comets (Oort cloud in the graph represents comets). The researchers came to a conclusion that Earth's water did not come from comets, but perhaps came from asteroids. However there are some other scientists and researchers who argue that our Earth got its water neither from comets not from asteroids.

The research findings of diverse studies are shown on the following chart.

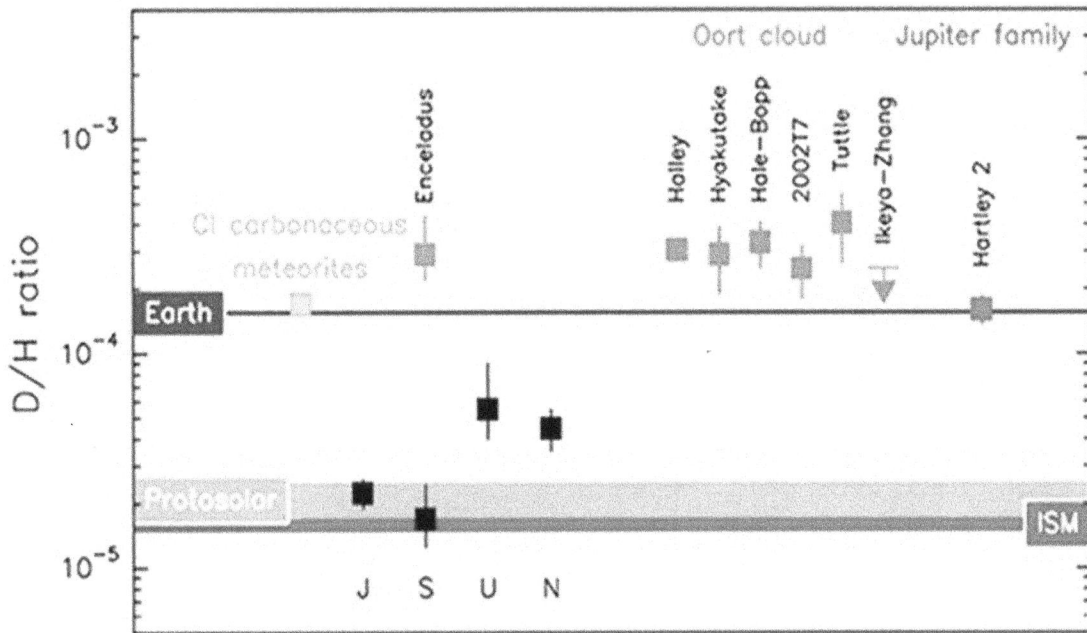

Courtesy of European Space Agency (ESA)
Figure 20.3 Comparison of D/H Ratios, the standard being the Earth's seawater.

EARTH WAS BOMBARDED BY COMETS AND ASTEROIDS [88, 89]

Our Solar System began its formation 6 billion years ago, and completed its formation 4.54 billion years ago. Our ancestors have been believing for centuries that about 4 to 3.8 billion years ago a period of intense comet and asteroid bombardment is thought to have peppered all the planets including the Earth. Many of the numerous craters (large bowl-shaped cavities in the ground) found by astronomers on the Moon and other bodies in the Solar System record this event.

One theory was: The giant planets Jupiter, Saturn, Uranus and Neptune migrated around the Solar System about 4 to 3.8 billion years ago, caused gravitational pulls, thereby slinging asteroids and comets toward the inner Solar System. The disrupted water-rich and ice-bearing comets and asteroids were blown in all directions and collided with the planets, including the Earth. The record of this exact occurrence and the pertinent details were lost on the Earth because our planet's tectonic plate system and active erosion that ensures that the Earth's surface is constantly renewed and recovered from the damage.

However some researchers found and recognized the asteroid impacts by examining the thick layers of rock droplets known as sand-sized spherules. By examining the thickness of the spherules, the researchers were able to determine the size of the asteroid, number of asteroids, number of impacts, and the approximate time of the impact in the history of the Earth. Some of the asteroids that they discovered were about 40 kilometers (24.8 miles) in diameter. The researchers estimated that approximately there were 70 hits by asteroids, much larger in size than those that killed dinosaurs, between 3.8 and 1.8 billion years ago. They also detected four other asteroid hits on the moon.

The researchers reported that the frequency of these impacts was high enough to reproduce the known spherule beds, and also hints at the possibility that two gigantic craters resulted from the Late Heavy Bombardment.

The Two Oldest and Biggests Asteroid Hits: (i) Nearly 112-mile-wide or 180-km-wide Vredefort crater (a large cavity deep into the Earth) in South Africa, which occurred 2 billion years ago, and (ii) Nearly 155-mile-wide or 250-km-wide Sudbury crater (another large cavity deep into the Earth) in Ontario, Canada, which occurred 1.85 billion years ago.

The researchers also believed that the asteroid impacts may have played a large role in the evolutional history of both animal and human life.

Asteroids currently are the most likely suspect for delivering water to the planet Earth. Astronomers and researchers believe from their research findings that small rocky bodies such as meteorites, more specifically carbonaceous chondrites, could have carried water and organic material during the late heavy bombardment as they constantly slammed onto the Earth's surface, causing the so-called "oceans."

Comets were eliminated from being a suspect for delivering water to the planet Earth, based on the the scientific research findings of water analysis (see below for more details).

THEORY # 1: COMMETS COUND HAVE BROUGHT WATER TO EARTH
Ia. RESEARCH FINDINGS ON COMETS
A Rare Case That Matched With Earth's Seawater [91, 92]

An Astronomy professor "Edwin (Ted) Bergin" of the University of Michigan, Ann Arbor, Michigan, USA along with his fellow researchers published a paper in 2011, matching the (D/H Ratio) of water from comets, for the first time, using the water sample obtained from the Herschel Space Observatory Jupiter-Family Comet 103P/Hartley 2.

Summary of their findings:
Earth's Oceans: 156 Deuterium atoms per 1 million atoms of Hydrogen
Therefore, D/H Ratio = 156×10^{-6} = 1.56×10^{-4}

Previously published measurements about water in 6 comets from the Oort cloud yielded
D/H Ratio = 296×10^{-6} = 2.96×10^{-4}
Which did not match with the D/H Ratio of Earth's seawater.

For Jupiter-Family Comet 103P/Hartley 2, Ted Bergin et al. obtained the following D/H Ratio.
D/H Ratio = 161×10^{-6} = 1.61×10^{-4}
Which is the only measurement found to be closest to the Earth's seawater.

Drawbacks of This Study: They obtained measurements for one small sample only. They did not confirm the result by repeating analysis of more samples to make sure that the value they calculated is indeed correct. They did not know if the comet is a representative member of the Kuiper Belt. Therefore the data and results of this study are not trustworthy. Based on this study alone, and based on the previously published information on comets, we cannot confirm that comets are the likely source of our Earth's seawater.
++

Journal Publication [92]
Ocean-like water in the **Jupiter-Family Comet 103P/Hartley 2**.

Authors: Paul Hartogh, Dariusz C. Lis, Dominique Bockelée-Morvan, Miguel de Val-Borro, Nicolas Biver, Michael Küppers, Martin Emprechtinger, Edwin A. Bergin, Jacques Crovisier, Miriam Rengel, Raphael Moreno, Slawomira Szutowicz & Geoffrey A. Blake,
Nature, Volume 478, pages 218–220, October 13, 2011.
https://www.nature.com/articles/nature10519

Abstract
For decades, the source of Earth's volatiles, especially water with a deuterium-to-hydrogen ratio (D/H) of $(1.558 \pm 0.001) \times 10-4$, has been a subject of debate. The similarity of Earth's bulk composition to that of meteorites known as enstatite chondrites suggests a dry proto-Earth2 with subsequent delivery of volatiles by local accretion or impacts of asteroids or comets. Previous measurements in six comets from the Oort cloud yielded a mean D/H ratio of $(2.96 \pm 0.25) \times 10-4$. The D/H value in carbonaceous chondrites, $(1.4 \pm 0.1) \times 10-4$, together with dynamical simulations, led to models in which asteroids were the main source of Earth's water, with ≤10 per cent being delivered by comets. Here we report that the D/H ratio in the Jupiter-family comet 103P/Hartley 2, which originated in the Kuiper belt, is $(1.61 \pm 0.24) \times 10-4$. This result substantially expands the reservoir of Earth ocean-like water to include some comets, and is consistent with the emerging picture of a complex dynamical evolution of the early Solar System.
++

Ib. RESEARCH FINDINGS ON COMETS (ROSETTA MISSION)
Comets Could Not Have Brought Water To Earth [93, 94, 95, 96, 97, 98]

The European Space Agency's Rosetta spacecraft has found the water vapour from its target comet to be significantly different to that found on Earth. This discovery fueled the debate on the origin of our planet's oceans. The Rosetta spacecraft followed a 10-year mission to catch a comet and land a probe on it. Launched in 2004, the spacecraft arrived at its target, Comet 67P/Churyumov-Gerasimenko, on August 6, 2014. Since August, the Rosetta probe has been orbiting Comet 67P/Churyumov-Gerasimenko, and on November 12, 2014, its lander, Philae, made a historic touchdown on the object's surface. Although the robot's batteries ran out soon after setting down, it gathered a wealth of scientific data, and the Rosetta "mothership" continues to analyse the wandering "ice mountain".

Prof. Kathrin Altwegg, from the University of Bern in Switzerland was the Rosina's principal investigator. They emphasized that the ratio between heavy and light water (D/H Ratio) is very characteristic. This ratio cannot be easily changed as it stays steady for a long time.

If we could compare the water in comets with the water we have on Earth, we can definitely say if the water on Earth is compatible with the water on comets. The research team got a water sample from the Rosetta spacecraft, analysed and reported the following results:

D/H Ratio for the Comet 67P/Churyumov-Gerasimenko = $5.3 \pm 0.7 \times 10{-4}$
This result is more than three times higher than that we already found for the Earth's seawater, which means that this kind of comet could not have brought water to the Earth.

Earth's Oceans Contain: 156 deuterium atoms per 1 million hydrogen atom.
Therefore, D/H Ratio = $156 \times 10{-6} = 1.56 \times 10{-4}$

Previously published measurements about water in 6 comets from the Oort cloud yielded
D/H Ratio = $296 \times 10{-6} = 2.96 \times 10{-4}$
Which did not match with the D/H Ratio of Earth's seawater at all.
++

Journal Publication: Rosetta Mission [98]

67P/Churyumov-Gerasimenko, a Jupiter family comet with a high D/H ratio
Authors: K. Altwegg1,*, H. Balsiger1, A. Bar-Nun2, J. J. Berthelier3, A. Bieler1,4,
P. Bochsler1, C. Briois5, U. Calmonte1, M. Combi4,
Science Vol. 347, Issue 6220, 1261952, Jan 23, 2015.
http://science.sciencemag.org/content/347/6220/1261952

Abstract

The provenance of water and organic compounds on Earth and other terrestrial planets has been discussed for a long time without reaching a consensus. One of the best means to distinguish between different scenarios is by determining the deuterium-to-hydrogen (D/H) ratios in the reservoirs for comets and Earth's oceans. Here, we report the direct in situ measurement of the D/H ratio in the Jupiter family comet 67P/Churyumov-Gerasimenko by the ROSINA mass spectrometer aboard the European Space Agency's Rosetta spacecraft, which is found to be $(5.3 \pm 0.7) \times 10^{-4}$—that is, approximately three times the terrestrial value. Previous cometary measurements and our new finding suggest a wide range of D/H ratios in the water within Jupiter family objects and preclude the idea that this reservoir is solely composed of Earth ocean–like water.

CONCLUSION

THEORY # 1 COMETS COULD HAVE BROUGHT WATER TO EARTH

The presumption that Comets could have brought water to our planet Earth was proved to be wrong based on the water analysis of water samples obtained from Comets. The European Space Agency's Rosetta spacecraft has found that the water vapour from its target comet to be significantly different to that found on Earth. The Deuterium-to-Hydrogen Ratio (D/H Ratio) of the water from the Comets was found to be a lot higher than that of sea water. Based on the aforementioned scientific measurements and calculations, the scientists concluded that the Earth's water could not have come from the Comets. However the analyses of more water samples from Comets are needed to confirm these findings.

THEORY # 2: ASTEROIDS COULD HAVE BROUGHT WATER TO EARTH
III. RESEARCH FINDINGS ON ASTEROIDS (Meteorites/Carbonaceous Chondrites)
[99, 100, 101, 102, 103, 104, 105, 106, 107, 108, 109, 110, 111, 112, 113, 114, 115, 116, 117, 118, 119]

NASA posted that there are more than 326 million trillion gallons of water on Earth. Earth's oceans contain about 96.5 percent of all the planet's water. Less than 3 percent of all water on Earth is freshwater (usable for drinking). More than two-thirds of Earth's freshwater is locked up in ice caps and glaciers. [80]

Big Bang started the energy that sparked the outward swelling of space transmuted into a hot, uniform and expanding bath of particles. One second after the Big Bang, our Universe was filled with neutrons, protons, electrons, anti-electrons, photons and neutrinos. During the first three minutes of our Universe, the light elements hydrogen and helium were born during a process known as Big Bang "nucleosynthesis". Thereafter, temperatures cooled down, and protons and neutrons collided to make deuterium, an isotope of hydrogen. Most of the deuterium combined to make more helium, and more lithium. Producing copious amounts of hydrogen is a propitious start en route to water, but the nature needs oxygen in order to form water (H_2O).

That's where "factories" called stars enter the picture, which manufactured oxygen in their burning cores. Deep within their blisteringly hot interiors, stars are nuclear furnaces that fuse the Big Bang's simple nuclei (hydrogen, helium and lithium) into more complex elements, including carbon, nitrogen, oxygen, and other elements we see in the periodic table today. Later in their lives, when stars exploded into supernovae, the explosions spew these elements into space. Oxygen and hydrogen commingle to make water (H_2O). We knew that the star (our Sun) began its formation from a supernova explosion of an earlier humongous star some 6 billion years ago. Water molecules were surely part of the dusty swirl that coalesced into the Sun and its surrounding 8 planets, along with comets and asteroids. But Earth's early history, including epochs with high ambient temperatures and no enveloping atmosphere, implies that surface water would have evaporated and drifted back into space. Faced with this conundrum, astronomers realized that there are two ready-made sources: comets and asteroids, the Solar System's gravel strewn among planetary boulders. The primary difference between the two is that comets typically have a greater concentration of ingredients that vaporize when heated, accounting for their iconic gaseous tails. Both comets and asteroids can contain ice. And if, by colliding with Earth, they added the amount of material some scientists suspect, such bodies could easily have delivered oceans' worth of water. Accordingly, each has been fingered as a suspect in the mystery of water on our planet Earth. [99]

Adjudicating between the comets and asteroids is a challenge, and over the years scientific judgment has swung from one to the other. Nevertheless, recent observations of their chemical makeups are tipping the scale toward asteroids. Researchers reported that the D/H Ratio in asteroids appear to better match with the water on Earth.

Asteroids are rocky fragments that orbit the Sun in a belt between Mars and Jupiter. Asteroids exist in different types. The main asteroid belt is located between about 2 and 3.2 Astronomical Units (AU). One Astronomical Unit is the Earth-Sun distance. The inner part of the main belt is dominated by S-type asteroids and the outer part by C-types.

We can use meteorites to figure out what asteroids are actually made of. Meteorites are pieces of asteroids that land on Earth. By determining what different types of meteorites would look like if they were floating around in space, we can figure out which meteorites go with which types of asteroids. It turns out that the inner part of the asteroid belt is drier and the outer part is wetter. S-type asteroids, associated with ordinary chondrite meteorites, are dry. C-type asteroids, associated with carbonaceous chondrite meteorites, are wet, with about 10% water by mass. [100]

When our Solar System was born, planets formed in giant frisbee-shaped disks (that look like flying saucers) around the young burning star, our Sun. Close to the Sun, the rocky planets (Mercury, Venus, Earth & Mars) orbit and these planets receive too much heat from the Sun so water existed in the form of vapour. Farther to the Sun, the giant, gassy and icy planets (Jupiter, Saturn, Uranus and Neptune) orbit in which water is condensed and form ice deposits. During the early stages of its formation, the rocky planet Earth could have received its water when the icy outer planets and asteroids (C-type meteorites) bashed the Earth. The researchers were able to find out the origin of water from water analysis and from the D/H Ratio.

Several researchers, after analysing the water samples from asteroids, meteorites, concluded that the Earth's water most likely accreted during the early stages of the rock formation. The planet Earth formed as a wet planet with water on the surface during the first million years. The relevant journal publications are given below:

++

Journal Publication [109]

Early accretion of water in the inner Solar System from a carbonaceous chondrite–like source. Authors: Adam R. Sarafian, Sune G. Nielsen, Horst R. Marschall, Francis M. McCubbin, Brian D. Monteleone.
Science, Vol. 346, Issue 6209, pp. 623-626, 31 Oct 2014.
http://science.sciencemag.org/content/346/6209/623

History Recorded In Asteroid's Water

Astronomers know that interstellar water is abundantly available to young planetary systems—our blue planet collected (or accreted) plenty of it. Still, the details of water's movement in the inner Solar System are elusive. Sarafian et al. measured water isotopes in meteorite samples from the asteroid Vesta for clues to the timing of water accretion. Their samples have the same isotopic fingerprint of volatiles as both Earth and carbonaceous chondrites, some of the most primitive meteorites. The findings suggest that Earth received most of its water relatively early from chondrite-like bodies.

Abstract

Determining the origin of water and the timing of its accretion within the inner Solar System is important for understanding the dynamics of planet formation. The timing of water accretion to the inner Solar System also has implications for how and when life emerged on Earth. We report in situ measurements of the hydrogen isotopic composition of the mineral apatite in eucrite meteorites, whose parent body is the main-belt asteroid 4 Vesta. These measurements sample one of the oldest hydrogen reservoirs in the Solar System and show that Vesta contains the same hydrogen isotopic composition as that of carbonaceous chondrites. Taking into account the old ages of eucrite meteorites and their similarity to Earth's isotopic ratios of hydrogen, carbon, and nitrogen, we demonstrate that these volatiles could have been added early to Earth, rather than gained during a late accretion event.

++

Journal Publication [112]
The Provenances of Asteroids, and Their Contributions to the Volatile Inventories of the Terrestrial Planets, Authors: C. M. O'D. Alexander1,*, R. Bowden2, M. L. Fogel2, K. T. Howard3,4, C. D. K. Herd5, L. R. Nittler1
Science, Vol. 337, Issue 6095, pp. 721-723, DOI: 10.1126/science.1223474, Aug 10, 2012.
http://science.sciencemag.org/content/337/6095/721.full?sid=aa2da622-520a-4813-b0b5-30bdc95f33bf

Constraining the Birthplace of Asteroids

Many primitive meteorites originating from the asteroid belt once contained abundant water that is now stored as OH in hydrated minerals. Alexander et al. (p. 721, published online 12 July) estimated the hydrogen isotopic compositions in 86 samples of primitive meteorites that fell in Antarctica and compared the results to those of comets and Saturn's moon, Enceladus. Water in primitive meteorites was less deuterium-rich than that in comets and Enceladus, implying that, in contradiction to recent models of the dynamical evolution of the Solar System, the parent bodies of primitive meteorites cannot have formed in the same region as comets. The results also suggest that comets were not the principal source of Earth's water.

Abstract

Determining the source(s) of hydrogen, carbon, and nitrogen accreted by Earth is important for understanding the origins of water and life and for constraining dynamical processes that operated during planet formation. Chondritic meteorites are asteroidal fragments that retain records of the first few million years of Solar System history. The deuterium/hydrogen (D/H Ratio) values of water in carbonaceous chondrites are distinct from those in comets and Saturn's moon Enceladus, implying that they formed in a different region of the Solar System, contrary to predictions of recent dynamical models. The D/H values of water in carbonaceous chondrites also argue against an influx of water ice from the outer Solar System, which has been invoked to explain the nonsolar oxygen isotopic composition of the inner Solar System. The bulk hydrogen and nitrogen isotopic compositions of CI chondrites suggest that they were the principal source of Earth's volatiles.
++

Journal Publication [114]
Vortex magnetic structure in framboidal magnetite reveals existence of water droplets in an ancient asteroid. Authors: Yuki Kimura, Takeshi Sato, Norihiro Nakamura, Jun Nozawa, Tomoki Nakamura, Katsuo Tsukamoto & Kazuo Yamamoto
Nature Communications volume 4, Article number: 2649, October 22, 2013.
https://www.nature.com/articles/ncomms3649

Abstract

The majority of water has vanished from modern meteorites, yet there remain signatures of water on ancient asteroids. How and when water disappeared from the asteroids is important, because the final fluid-concentrated chemical species played critical roles in the early evolution of organics and in the final minerals in meteorites. Here we show evidence of vestigial traces of water based on a nanometre-scale palaeomagnetic method, applying electron holography to the framboids in the Tagish Lake meteorite. The framboids are colloidal crystals composed of three-dimensionally ordered magnetite nanoparticles and therefore are only able to form against the repulsive force induced by the surface charge of the magnetite as a water droplet parches in microgravity. We demonstrate that the magnetites have a flux closure vortex structure, a unique magnetic configuration in nature that permits the formation of colloidal crystals just before exhaustion of water from a local system within a hydrous asteroid.
++

+++

Journal Publication [115]

A dual origin for water in carbonaceous asteroids revealed by CM chondrites.

Authors: Laurette Piani, Hisayoshi Yurimoto & Laurent Remusat

Nature Astronomy, Volume 2, Pages 317–323, March 12, 2018.
https://www.nature.com/articles/s41550-018-0413-4

Abstract

Carbonaceous asteroids represent the principal source of water in the inner Solar System and might correspond to the main contributors for the delivery of water to Earth. Hydrogen isotopes in water-bearing primitive meteorites, for example carbonaceous chondrites, constitute a unique tool for deciphering the sources of water reservoirs at the time of asteroid formation. However, fine-scale isotopic measurements are required to unravel the effects of parent-body processes on the pre-accretion isotopic distributions. Here, we report in situ micrometre-scale analyses of hydrogen isotopes in six CM-type carbonaceous chondrites, revealing a dominant deuterium-poor water component mixed with deuterium-rich organic matter. We suggest that this deuterium-poor water corresponds to a ubiquitous water reservoir in the inner protoplanetary disk. A deuterium-rich water signature has been preserved in the least altered part of the Paris chondrite in hydrated phases possibly present in the CM rock before alteration. The presence of the deuterium-enriched water signature in Paris might indicate that transfers of ice from the outer to the inner Solar System were significant within the first million years of the history of the Solar System.

+++

Journal Publication [118]

https://arxiv.org/abs/1707.01234

Origin of water in the inner Solar System: Planetesimals scattered inward during Jupiter and Saturn's rapid gas accretion.

Authors: Sean N. Raymond, Andre Izidoro

Icarus, 297, 134-148 (2017), DOI: 10.1016/j.icarus.2017.06.030

Abstract

There is a long-standing debate regarding the origin of the terrestrial planets' water as well as the hydrated C-type asteroids. Here we show that the inner Solar System's water is a simple byproduct of the giant planets' formation. Giant planet cores accrete gas slowly until the conditions are met for a rapid phase of runaway growth. As a gas giant's mass rapidly increases, the orbits of nearby planetesimals are destabilized and gravitationally scattered in all directions. Under the action of aerodynamic gas drag, a fraction of scattered planetesimals are deposited onto stable orbits interior to Jupiter's. This process is effective in populating the outer main belt with C-type asteroids that originated from a broad (5-20 AU-wide) region of the disk. As the disk starts to dissipate, scattered planetesimals reach sufficiently eccentric orbits to cross the terrestrial planet region and deliver water to the growing Earth. This mechanism does not depend strongly on the giant planets' orbital migration history and is generic: whenever a giant planet forms it invariably pollutes its inner planetary system with water-rich bodies.

+++

CONCLUSION

THEORY # 2 ASTEROIDS COULD HAVE BROUGHT WATER TO EARTH

The presumption that Asteroids could have brought water to our planet Earth was investigated by many researchers. When our Solar System was born, planets formed around the young burning star, our Sun. Close to the burning Sun, the rocky planets (Mercury, Venus, Earth & Mars) orbit and these planets receive too much heat from the Sun so water existed in the form of vapour. Farther to the Sun, the giant, gassy and icy planets (Jupiter, Saturn, Uranus and Neptune) orbit in which water is condensed and form ice deposits. During the early stages of its formation, the rocky planet Earth could have received its water when the icy outer planets and asteroids (C-type meteorites) bashed the Earth. The researchers were able to match the Deuterium-to-Hydrogen Ratio (D/H Ratio) between the sea water and the water samples from Asteroids. Which means the Earth could have accreted up to 50% of its water from Asteroids during the early states after its formation.

However many readers might be having a lingering question such as **"How did those Asteroids get their water?"**

Dr. RK provided the following answer: After all, those Asteroids are part of our Solar System. Water formation took place in the interstellar medium even before the formation of our Solar System (before 6 billion years ago). Our Earth, Asteroids, Comets, and other 7 planets belong to our Solar System. All of them got their water even before the formation of our Solar System from a star-forming cloud (which became our Solar System) in the interstellar medium where the abundantly available hydrogen and oxygen commingled under the appropriate climate conditions by the chemical reaction $2 H_2 + O_2 = 2 H_2O$, and formed ice-cold water molecules. Those ice-cold water molecules then entered into the space dust (also known as stardust) and interstellar gas in the interstellar medium, from a gigantic cloud of which our Solar System was created. Whatever water our Solar System possessed now was originally created in the star-forming cloud in the interstellar medium. You will learn more about the interstellar medium, and formation of water in the interstellar medium in the next section THEORY # 3. Please read THEORY # 3 for more information.

THEORY # 3: EARTH INHERITED ITS WATER FROM THE INTERSTELLAR MEDIUM EVEN BEFORE OUR SOLAR SYSTEM WAS BORN

It is now time to understand what "the interstellar medium" is all about.

INTERSTELLAR MEDIAN OR INTERSTELLAR SPACE
[120, 121, 122, 123, 124, 125, 126, 127, 128]

• The interstellar medium (ISM) or interstellar space is the material found between two stars, among three or more stars or amid many stars. It looks mostly like an empty space within a galaxy, filled with energy, in the form of electromagnetic radiation.

• The early massive first generation stars had very short lifetimes and ended in type II supernovae spreading their fused and remaining unfused molecules into the material occupying the gaps between or among the stars known as the interstellar medium (ISM). [73]

• The interstellar medium is mainly made up of gas (99%) with some dust (1%) and some cosmic rays. The gas exists in the ionic, atomic, and molecular form. The gas is mostly hydrogen (90%), with a little helium (9%), and small amounts of heavier elements such as carbon, nitrogen and oxygen (1%). The material or matter fills the interstellar space and blends smoothly into the surrounding intergalactic space. The interstellar medium has an extremely low density, so low that the gas around our Solar System contains only one atom in ten cubic centimeters (although there are regions with higher densities like "nebulas" that have millions of atoms per cubic centimetre). A nebula is nothing but a huge cloud of dust and gas mixed and coalesced with the leftovers of a previous star upon death. The dust particles are extremely small, and consist of silicates, carbon, ice, and/or iron compounds.

• The interstellar medium (ISM) is the birth place of stars. Stars form within the densest regions of the ISM, molecular clouds, and replenish the ISM with matter and energy through planetary nebulae (huge clouds of gas and dust), stellar winds, and supernova explosions.

• The dust, which makes up about 1% in the interstellar medium, is made of thin, highly flattened flakes or needles of graphite (carbon) and silicates (rock-like minerals) coated with water ice. Each dust flake is roughly the size of the wavelength of blue light or smaller. The dust is probably formed in the cool outer layers of red giant stars and dispersed in the red giant winds and planetary nebulae. [127]

• Scientists define the beginning of the interstellar space as the place where the Sun's constant flow of material and magnetic field stop affecting its surroundings. This place is called the heliopause. It marks the end of a region created by our Sun that is called the heliosphere. The Sun creates this heliosphere by sending a constant flow of particles and a magnetic field out into space at over 670,000 miles per hour. This stream is called the 'solar wind.' Once you arrive in the interstellar space, there would be an increase of "cold" particles around you. There would also be a magnetic field that does not originate from our Sun.

• The primordial matter produced in the Big Bang was almost entirely hydrogen and helium, with trace amounts of lithium, beryllium, and boron. There were no heavier elements (especially there was no oxygen yet) until the first star was born after 380,000 years. The first stars that formed in our Universe and in our Milky Way galaxy were made up of only these light elements. These stars were very massive, and had very short lifespans compared to many of the stars today. These stars continually fused the atoms of the lighter elements together to create the heavier elements such as carbon, nitrogen, oxygen, and the rest of the elements that we see in the periodic table today. When these stars died later with supernova explosions, the elements such as metals and minerals (silicon, iron, cobalt, uranium, and all others) were formed, and new material, consisting of more new elements, is recycled back into the interstellar space. The interstellar medium thereafter became enriched with the diverse elements needed for the evolution of new stars and planets such as our Sun and our Earth, and even the life formation. The gravity pulled the interstellar medium together to form newer stars and the surrounding planets.

⦿ All the atoms of our planet Earth such as carbon, oxygen, nitrogen, etc. (except hydrogen which is the only primordial element), and more specifically all the atoms of our bodies, were all produced in the burning cores of ancient stars which have been perished long ago after scattering fractions or all of their constituents to the interstellar medium (ISM). After all, aren't we all made up of mostly stardust? [128]

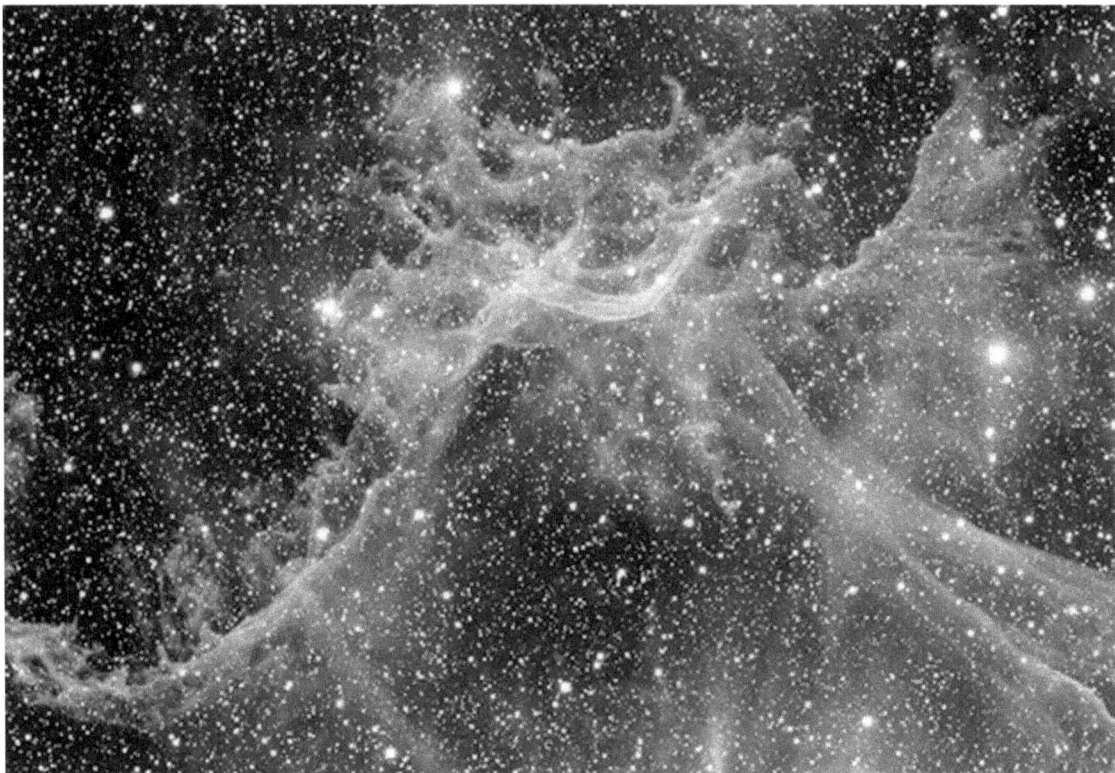

Courtesy of NASA.
Figure 20.4 The picture of the interstellar medium.
Our Solar System began its formation some 6 billion years ago from a solar nebula of space dust (also called stardust) and the interstellar gas in the interstellar medium.

WATER FOUND IN THE INTERSTELLAR MEDIUM (ISM) [129, 130]
A team of American astronomers, led by Cornell University astrophysicist Martin Harwit, has discovered a massive concentration of water vapor within a cloud of the interstellar gas close to the Orion nebula. The amount of water measured is so high -- enough to fill the Earth's oceans 60 times a day -- that the researchers believe it provides an important clue to the origin of water in the Solar System, and on our planet Earth.

The amount of water vapor measured in Orion is 20 times larger than that observed in other interstellar gas clouds in our Milky Way Galaxy. The measurements were made with the long-wavelength spectrometer aboard the Infrared Space Observatory (ISO) launched in November 1995 by the European Space Agency with the participation of NASA. The observations were made in October 1997, and reported later in the Astrophysical Journal Letters. The interstellar gas cloud that they observed was being pummelled by shock waves that compress and heat the gas. These shock waves were the result of the violent early stages of starbirth upon supernova explosion, in which a young star spews out gas that slams into its surroundings at high speed. The heated water vapour that they observed was believed to be the result of that collision.

The interstellar gas cloud that they observed in Orion seemed to be a huge chemical factory, capable to generate enough water molecules to fill over the Earth's oceans 60 times in a single day. Eventually that water vapour would cool and freeze, turning into small solid particles of ice. Similar ice particles were presumably present within the gas cloud from which the Solar System originally formed. It seemed quite plausible that much of the water in our Solar System was originally produced in a giant water-vapour factory like the one they observed in Orion.

How Did the Water Get Into The Interstellar Medium?

Nearly 380,000 years after the Big Bang, hydrogen was first created, and thereafter it was readily available throughout our Universe. Nearly 400 million years after the Big Bang, stars formation commenced using hydrogen as the burning fuel. The massive pressure build-up of the fiery inferno within the stars was so great that hydrogen atoms fused together to form heavier element helium, and helium atoms in turn fused together to form much heavier elements such as lithium, beryllium, carbon, nitrogen, oxygen, and others in a process known as "**stellar nucleosynthesis.**" The early stars were massive and short-lived. When the massive stars finished burning their hydrogen or helium fuel, they eventually extinguished, collapsed as they could not withstand their own gravitational force, and exploded into supernovae while dumping and scattering all kinds of heavier elements (the most important are carbon, nitrogen, oxygen, phosphorus and sulfur and others) across the interstellar medium of our Milky Way Galaxy, and also across the other galaxies our Universe.

More than 6 billion years ago, during the supernova explosions in our Milky Way Galaxy, those newly formed heavier elements, including the very important oxygen, commingled together and formed all kinds of newer elements that we see in our periodic table today (there are 117 heavier elements). Space scientists discovered that when newer elements were being formed, the abundantly available hydrogen and oxygen commingled together and formed water molecules by the chemical reaction ($2 H_2 + O_2 = 2 H_2O$). Those water molecules then entered into the space dust and interstellar gas in the interstellar medium, from a gigantic cloud of which our Solar System (our Sun, our Earth, our Moon & 7 other planets) was created. And that is how our Earth inherited liquid water 6 billion years ago even before it was born. The formation of our Solar System completed 4.54 billion years ago, and our Earth was thus born with water.

The intriguing idea is that the ice-cold water from the interstellar medium was incorporated with a lot of organic material in it, which could have helped kick-start the life on our planet Earth.

The icy coating is built up on the dust grains over time. Water is therefore deposited in the form of icy coating on the dust particles. These molecules of water leave the clouds of gas and dust and end up in many different places – planets, comets, asteroids and the centers of galaxies. Milky Way Galaxy is where our Solar System is located. This is how our planet Earth accreted water from the interstellar space. Scientists believe that our planet Earth was originally born wet with plenty of water, and the belief that comets brought water to our planet Earth was later proved to be a myth.

IIIa. RESEARCH FINDINGS ON WATER FORMATION [134, 135]
INTERSTELLAR MEDIUM IS WHERE WATER FORMATION OCCURRED

Since our Solar System evolved from an interstellar molecular cloud, it was reported by several astronomers and scientists that icy objects in the Solar System originated from the water ice formed in the interstellar molecular cloud.

A team of Japanese researchers shed light on those revelations on water formation in the interstellar medium through conducting a laboratory research project. The purpose of the research project was to gain an understanding of the origin of water molecules in interstellar clouds. After a thorough review of the published literature on the interstellar medium, the research group has concluded that water must form when atomic hydrogen interacts with frozen solid oxygen on a solid surface, such as dust grains in interstellar clouds.

They therefore created a model laboratory setup for the first time with the conditions similar to interstellar space. They recreated this process by creating a layer of solid oxygen on an aluminum substrate, a metallic base, at a very cold temperature of -263 degrees Celcius (Absolute temperature = -263 degrees Celcius + 273 = 10 degrees Kelvin = 10 °K) and then exposed the cold surface to atomic hydrogen. With the infrared spectroscopy measurements, they confirmed that both water (H_2O) and hydrogen peroxide (H_2O_2) formed in the significant quantities, which explains the abundance of water formation seen in interstellar clouds.

It's interesting to note from this experiment that the first water molecules in our Universe must have started in this way. Those water molecules from the dust particles of the interstellar medium eventually ended up on the planet Earth, causing the life formation, and then eventually the Earth was populated by 7 billion people.

They then published their scientific findings in The Astrophysical Journa shown below: Some other researchers also published similar research findings (see below).

+++

Journal Publication [135]

Water Formation through a Quantum Tunneling Surface Reaction, OH + H_2, at 10 °K.
Authors: Oba, Y.; Watanabe, N.; Hama, T.; Kuwahata, K.; Hidaka, H.; and Kouchi, A.
The Astrophysical Journal, Volume 749, Issue 1, article id. 67, 12 pp. (2012).
(ApJ Homepage), Publication Date: April 2012.
http://adsabs.harvard.edu/abs/2012ApJ...749...67O

Abstract
The present study experimentally demonstrated that solid H_2O is formed through the surface reaction OH + H_2 at 10 K. This is the first experimental evidence of solid H_2O formation using hydrogen in its molecular form at temperatures as low as 10 °K. We further found that H_2O formation through the reaction OH + H_2 is about one order of magnitude more effective than HDO formation through the reaction OH + D_2. This significant isotope effect results from differences in the effective mass of each reaction, indicating that the reactions proceed through quantum tunneling.

+++

++

Journal Publication [136]

Experimental evidence for water formation on interstellar dust grains by hydrogen and oxygen atoms. Authors: F. Dulieu, L. Amiaud, E. Congiu, J-H. Fillion, E. Matar, A. Momeni, V. Pirronello, J. L. Lemaire.
Journal of Astronmy & Astrophysics, Volume 512, March-April 2010.
https://www.aanda.org/articles/aa/full_html/2010/04/aa12079-09/aa12079-09.html

Complete Paper, PDF File
https://www.aanda.org/articles/aa/pdf/2010/04/aa12079-09.pdf

Context: The synthesis of water is one necessary step in the origin and development of life. It is believed that pristine water is formed and grows on the surface of icy dust grains in dark interstellar clouds. Until now, there has been no experimental evidence whether this scenario is feasible or not on an astrophysically relevant template and by hydrogen and oxygen atom reactions.

Aims: We present here the first experimental evidence of water synthesis by such a process on a realistic grain surface analogue in dense clouds, i.e., amorphous water ice.

Methods: Atomic beams of oxygen and deuterium are aimed at a porous water ice substrate (H_2O) held at 10 °K. Products are analyzed by the temperature-programmed desorption technique.

Results: We observe production of Hydrogen-deuterium oxide (HDO) and Deuterium oxide (D_2O), indicating that water is formed under conditions of the dense interstellar medium from hydrogen and oxygen atoms. This experiment opens up the field of a little explored complex chemistry that could occur on dust grains, believed to be the site where key processes lead to the molecular diversity and complexity observed in our Universe.
++

Journal Publication [138]

ON WATER FORMATION IN THE INTERSTELLAR MEDIUM: LABORATORY STUDY OF THE O+D REACTION ON SURFACES, Authors: Dapeng Jing, Jiao He, John Brucato, Antonio De Sio, Lorenzo Tozzetti, and Gianfranco Vidali, The American Astronomical Society.
The Astrophysical Journal Letters, Volume 741, Number 1, October 10 2011.
http://iopscience.iop.org/article/10.1088/2041-8205/741/1/L9

Abstract

In the interstellar medium (ISM), an important channel of water formation is the reaction of atoms on the surface of dust grains. Here, we report on a laboratory study of the formation of water via the O+D reaction network. While prior studies were done on ices, as appropriate to the formation of water in dense clouds, we explored how water formation occurs on bare surfaces, i.e., in conditions mimicking the transition from diffuse to dense clouds (Av ~ 1-5). Reaction products were detected during deposition and afterward when the sample is brought to a high temperature. We quantified the formation of water and intermediary products, such as hydrogen peroxide D_2O_2, over a range of surface temperatures (15-25 K). The detection of OD on the surface signals the importance of this reactant in the overall scheme of water formation in the ISM.
++

IIIb. RESEARCH FINDINGS ON WATER FORMATION
EARTH INHERITED ITS WATER FROM THE INTERSTELLAR MEDIUM
THE WATER THAT YOU DRINK TODAY IS OLDER THAN 4.54 Billion Years!
[139, 140, 141, 142, 143, 144, 145, 146, 147, 148]

Water is known to form in the clouds of gas and dust of the interstellar medium (ISM). It is also known that the gas and dust particles then coalesce and form planetary systems, but the water is most likely destroyed when the newly formed Sun starts pumping out heat and light. Astronomers believed for decades that water on Earth formed again later from the aid of comets and asteroids. But a recent study shed new light on the water formation, as a new research team proved that primordial water survived within the Earth even before Solar System was formed. That means the water you drink today is much older than 4.54 billion years.

A PhD student, Ms. Ilsedore Cleeves, from the Department of Astronomy, University of Michigan, Ann Arbor, Michigan, USA, developed a doctoral thesis, and her thesis was approved based on the conclusion that the Earth inherited up to 50% of its water from the interstellar medium, water was not completely evaporated after our Sun was born, but remained hidden within the dust particles until and after the formation of the Earth. She, her supervisor, and fellow researchers published a paper in the Science journal in 2014.

Mathematical Modeling & Simulation: The research team constructed a detailed mathematical model of the water-forming chemical processes, including the best basic principles and laws of physics and chemistry known to astronomers, physicists and chemists today. The mathematical model was so powerful that it could predict the amount of deuterium and deuterium-hydrogen ratio (D/H Ratio) at any desired time once the coalescence of gas and dust particles began and protoplanetary disc began its formation. Much of the cosmic rays are fended off by the young star's magnetic field and particles streaming out from the star, but there are other sources of radiation: X-rays from the star and short-lived radionuclides in the disk. The frozen water formation requires the colder temperatures from 263.15 to -243.15 Celsius (10 to 30 degrees Kelvin) of in order to takes place the appropriate reactions. The model was verified by using the real-time data of Earth's seawater, water from comets and asteroids (meteorites). The researchers were fully satisfied by the powerful predictions the mathematical model has been delivering.

The Results: They reset the parameters to the beginning of the Solar System (our Solar System was born 4.54 billion years ago), and simulated the protoplanetary disc without frozen heavy eater (heavy water means deuterium-enriched water). Protoplanetary disk is a disk of gas and dust, often geometrically thin and opaque, orbiting a newly formed star (our Sun), from which planets including our Earth eventually form. They allowed the Solar System to make water from scratch on its own, and monitored the dynamic behaviour of the Deuterium and D/H Ratio in the water continuously for 1 million years, which is the standard timeframe required for formation of planets in a Solar System. They discovered that the system could not produce deuterium-rich water and could not achieve the D/H Ratio usually found in the samples of water from comets, meteorites and Earth's oceans.

IMPORTANT RESEARCH FINDINGS: The simulation results showed that a significant amount of water, the most-fundamental ingredient to fostering life, was not made in the protoplanetary disk of the Solar System. Instead, the Earth inherited its water from the interstellar medium, meaning that the water that is available on our Earth is older than our Sun (the formation of our Sun began 6 billion years ago, and its formation completed 4.54 billion years ago).

The results also showed that as much as 50% of the water now on Earth may have existed since before the birth of the Sun, 4.54 billion years ago. And that's good news for other planetary systems. The conditions in the ISM are far more uniform across space than those in protoplanetary disks, so it's likely that there is water everywhere waiting for planets to form. So the availability of water and the formation of life is possible in many other planets out there in our Milky Way Galaxy as the interstellar space has identical characteristics.

Bottom Line: A researcher in her doctoral thesis in the department of astronomy, University of Michigan, Ann Arbor, Michigan, USA concluded that up to 50% of the water on Earth is likely older than the Solar System itself. Much of the water on Earth and throughout our Solar System likely originated as ice deposited on the dust particles that formed in interstellar space. The remaining 50% of the water might have resulted from the bombardment of asteroids (meteorites). The intriguing idea is that the ices from the interstellar medium were incorporated with a lot of organic material in them, which could have helped kick-start the life on Earth.

Dr. Ilsedore Cleeves published a paper in 2014 in the Science journal along with other contributors Dr. Edwin (Ted) Bergin, Professor and Chair, Department of Astronomy, University of Michigan, Ann Arbor, Michigan, USA, Dr. Conel Alexander, Department of Terrestrial Magnetism, Carnegie Institution of Washington, Washington, DC 20015, USA, and several other researchers. The details of the publication are given below:

++
Journal Publication [148]
Publication Title: The ancient heritage of water ice in the Solar System.
Authors: L. Ilsedore Cleeves, Edwin (Ted) A. Bergin, Conel M. O'D. Alexander, Fujun Du, Dawn Graninger, Karin I. Öberg, Tim J. Harries, University of Michigan, Carnegie DTM Harvard-Smithsonian CfA, University of Exeter.
Science, Vol. 345 no. 6204 pp. 1590-1593, Submitted on 25 Sep 2014, Published in 2014.
https://arxiv.org/abs/1409.7398

Abstract
Identifying the source of Earth's water is central to understanding the origins of life-fostering environments and to assessing the prevalence of such environments in space. Water throughout the Solar System exhibits deuterium-to-hydrogen enrichments, a fossil relic of low-temperature, ion-derived chemistry within either (i) the parent molecular cloud or (ii) the solar nebula protoplanetary disk. Utilizing a comprehensive treatment of disk ionization, we find that ion-driven deuterium pathways are inefficient, curtailing the disk's deuterated water formation and its viability as the sole source for the Solar System's water. This finding implies that if the Solar System's formation was typical, abundant interstellar ices are available to all nascent planetary systems.

++

IIc. RESEARCH FINDINGS ON WATER FORMATION
EARTH GOT ITS WATER EVEN BEFORE THE MOON FORMATION [149, 150]

Previously it was thought that most, or even all, of Earth's ocean water was carried to the planet by comets and/or asteroids after the moon was formed. But according to the research findings of Dr. Richard Greenwood and his colleagues at the Open University in Milton Keynes, UK, our planet Earth might have had lakes and oceans even before the occurrence of a giant impact that created the moon.

Dr. Greenwood and his colleagues compared the oxygen composition of moon rocks brought back to Earth by Apollo astronauts with that of volcanic rocks from the ocean floor. The presence of liquid water alters the amounts of different oxygen isotopes in the rock. So, if most of the water on Earth had arrived after the giant impact, the rocks should have distinctly different oxygen compositions. The moon rocks should show little sign of being altered by water. The researchers found that most of the water we have now may have already been here 4.54 billion years ago or much earlier. They concluded that between about 5% and 30% of the Earth's water was brought later by asteroids and/or comets. They published their research findings in a journal paper shown below.

++
Journal Publication [150]
Oxygen isotopic evidence for accretion of Earth's water before a high-energy Moon-forming giant impact. Authors: Richard C. Greenwood, Jean-Alix Barrat, Martin F. Miller, Mahesh Anand, Nicolas Dauphas, Ian A. Franchi, Patrick Sillard and Natalie A. Starkey.
Science Advances, Vol. 4, no. 3, eaao5928, DOI: 10.1126/sciadv.aao5928, 28 Mar 2018.
http://advances.sciencemag.org/content/4/3/eaao5928.full

Abstract
The Earth-Moon system likely formed as a result of a collision between two large planetary objects. Debate about their relative masses, the impact energy involved, and the extent of isotopic homogenization continues. We present the results of a high-precision oxygen isotope study of an extensive suite of lunar and terrestrial samples. We demonstrate that lunar rocks and terrestrial basalts show a 3 to 4 ppm (parts per million), statistically resolvable, difference in $\Delta^{17}O$. Taking aubrite meteorites as a candidate impactor material, we show that the giant impact scenario involved nearly complete mixing between the target and impactor. Alternatively, the degree of similarity between the $\Delta^{17}O$ values of the impactor and the proto-Earth must have been significantly closer than that between Earth and aubrites. If the Earth-Moon system evolved from an initially highly vaporized and isotopically homogenized state, as indicated by recent dynamical models, then the terrestrial basalt-lunar oxygen isotope difference detected by our study may be a reflection of post–giant impact additions to Earth. On the basis of this assumption, our data indicate that post–giant impact additions to Earth could have contributed between 5 and 30% of Earth's water, depending on global water estimates. Consequently, our data indicate that the bulk of Earth's water was accreted before the giant impact and not later, as often proposed.

++

CONCLUSION

THEORY # 3 EARTH INHERITED ITS WATER FROM THE INTERSTELLAR MEDIUM

A PhD thesis in the Department of Astronomy, University of Michigan, Ann Arbor, Michigan, USA was approved based on the conclusion that our planet Earth inherited up to 50% of its water from the interstellar medium even before our Solar System (our Sun, our Earth and other 7 planets) was formed. Much of the water on Earth and throughout our Solar System likely originated as ice deposited on the dust particles that formed in interstellar space. The remaining 50% of the water might have resulted from the bombardment of asteroids (meteorites) during or after early stages of our Earth formation. The intriguing idea is that the ices from the interstellar medium were incorporated with a lot of organic material in them, which could have helped kick-start the life on Earth. After this research publication in 2014, many journalists and health writers wrote articles on the Internet and on the newspapers confirming that "the water we drink today is older than 4.54 billion years (older than our Solar System)".

THEORY # 4 EARTH'S DEEP MANTLE HAS THE WATER FROM THE INTERSTELLAR MEDIUM

IV. EVIDENCE OF PRIMORDIAL WATER FOUND IN EARTH'S DEEP MANTLE THIS MAY BE THE MOST IMPORTANT DISCOVERY YET!
[151, 152, 153, 154, 155, 156, 157, 158, 159]

The University of Hawaii researchers shed new light on the origin of Earth's water. A new study demonstrated that Earth's oceans are as old as the Earth itself. The study uncovers the fact that the Earth's oceans are local, and more interestingly the assumptions of many astronomers that the Earth's oceans might have been filled by the bombardment of comets and/or asteroids have been challenged. The researchers found evidence for primordial water in Earth's deep mantle. The research team was led by a cosmochemist Dr. Lydia Hallis, then a postdoctoral fellow at the NASA Astrobiology Institute (UHNAI), University of Hawaii, Honolulu, Hawaii, USA and now Marie Curie Research Fellow at the University of Glasgow, Scotland.

The researchers collected samples of primitive rocks from the Baffin Island, Nunavut Territory, Canada back in 1985. The rock was believed to have been from the Earth's deep mantle and untouched since it came into existence during the formation of our planet Earth. After collecting those rocks, scientists have had a lot of time to analyze them in the intervening years. As a result of their efforts, we know that they contain a component from Earth's deep mantle.

On studying those rocks, the researchers found that the water contained in those primitive rocks of the Earth's deep mantle was normal water, but not heavy water, like the ones found in comets and asteroids (meteorites). The ion-microprobe instrumentation allowed the researchers to focus on minute pockets of glass inside these scientifically important rocks, and to detect the tiny amounts of water within. By studying the ratio of hydrogen to deuterium (D/H ratio) in the water provided them with valuable new clues as to its origins.

The following information is known to astronomers and scientists throughout the world: Earth's Oceans contain: 156 Deuterium atoms per 1 million atoms of Hydrogen.
Therefore for Earth's Oceans, D/H Ratio = $156 \times 10^{-6} = 1.56 \times 10^{-4}$

The researchers in the current study found that the D/H Ratio for the primitive rock from the Baffin Island, Nunavut Territory, Canada is a lot less than 1.56×10^{-4} indicating the fact that the water in the Earth's deep mantle is not deuterium-enriched, and so the water must have been inherited from the "interstellar medium" and survived in the deep mantle.

This discovery strongly suggested that water was present on Earth from the onset of its formation. In fact, researchers believe that water molecules were present in the stardust that circulated around the Sun as a disk for millions of years before completing its formation of the Earth. Over time these water-rich dust particles were drawn together to form our planet Earth. While quite a drastic amount of water got evaporated from the heat produced by the Sun in making of our planet, enough water survived on the Earth to form the water bodies. Later, however heavy water got added to the Earth's oceans from subsequent bombardments from wet comets and/or asteroids (meteorites) that are believed to have originated about the same time as the Earth. These icy bodies could have later enriched our Earth's oceans with Deuterium. The original water that is still hidden in the Earth's mantle is not deuterium enriched. This suggests another important fact that Earth could have had water and life even without any help from comets and/or asteroids (meteorites).

Dr. Lydia J. Hallis published a paper along with her fellow-researchers and supervisors. Dr. Gary Huss, Dr. Kazuhide Nagashima, and Prof. G. Jeffrey Taylor of the Hawaii Institute of Geophysics and Planetology, and Prof. Mike Mottl of the Department of Oceanography, Dr. Sæmundur A. Halldórsson, and Dr. David R. Hilton. The journal publication is shown below:

++

Journal Publication [159]

Evidence for primordial water in Earth's deep mantle.
Authors: Lydia J. Hallis, Gary R. Huss, Kazuhide Nagashima, G. Jeffrey Taylor, Sæmundur A. Halldórsson, David R. Hilton, Michael J. Mottl.
Science, Vol. 350, Issue 6262, pp. 795-797, 13 Nov 2015.
http://science.sciencemag.org/content/350/6262/795

https://www.researchgate.net/publication/283752386_Evidence_for_primordial_water_in_E arth%27s_deep_mantle

Shaking Out Water's Dusty Origin

Where did Earth's water come from? Lavas erupting on Baffin Island, Nunavut Territory, Canada, tap a part of Earth's mantle isolated from convective mixing. Lydia Hallis et al. studied hydrogen isotopes in the lavas that help to "fingerprint" the origin of water from what could be a primordial reservoir. The isotope ratios (D/H ratios) for the Baffin Island basalt lavas suggest a pre-solar origin of water in Earth, probably delivered by adsorption onto dust grains.

Abstract

The hydrogen-isotope deuterium-hydrogen ratio (D/H ratio) of Earth can be used to constrain the origin of its water. However, the most accessible reservoir, Earth's oceans, may no longer represent the original (primordial) D/H ratio, owing to changes caused by water cycling between the surface and the interior. Thus, a reservoir completely isolated from surface processes is required to define Earth's original D/H signature. Here we present data for Baffin Island and Icelandic lavas, which suggest that the deep mantle has a low D/H ratio (δD more negative than −218 per mil). Such strongly negative values indicate the existence of a component within Earth's interior that inherited its D/H ratio directly from the protosolar nebula.

++

IVb. RESEARCH FINDINGS ON WATER FORMATION
THERE IS AS MUCH WATER IN EARTH'S DEEP MANTLE AS IN ALL OCEANS
[160, 161]

Dr. Hongzhan Fei, PhD at the University of Bayreuth in Germany conducted some research to find out the amount of water in the rocks of deep Earth mantle. The research revealed that the deep Earth mantle holds about the same amount of water as our oceans possess currently. He also concluded that there is a global buffer layer 410 to 660 kilometres beneath us that separates the upper mantle from the lower mantle.

There seems to be a mounting evidence that there is much more water than expected beneath us, mostly locked up within the crystals of minerals as ions rather than liquid water. At least one team has previously discovered water-rich rock fragments in volcanic debris originating from the mantle. The research also suggesting that the water in these mantle depths was formed here on Earth rather than being delivered by comets and/or asteroids. They conducted laboratory experiments on synthetic rocks used to model those typically found in that layer, as well as the one below. The experiments on synthetic rocks revealed that the high water content throughout the mantle transition zone. Real-world geophysical and seismic measurements revealed that the viscosity of the mantle transition zone is lower than that of the upper mantle above and the lower mantle below, which extends as deep as 2900 kilometres. Dr. Hongzhan Fei along with his fellow researchers published a paper, shown below.

Dr. Steven Jacobsen of Northwestern University in Illinois, Evanston, Illinois, USA also believes that there is a vast amount of water locked inside rocks of the deep region of the mantle since solidification of the mantle. Also Dr. Graham Pearson at the University of Alberta, Edmonton, Alberta, Canada worked on this field and expressed his view positively. His research revealed that from the laboratory and field observations via geophysics and natural studies indicate that the mantle transition zone is likely to host significant amount of water.
++

Journal Publication [161]

A nearly water-saturated mantle transition zone inferred from mineral viscosity.
Authors: Hongzhan Fei, Daisuke Yamazaki, Moe Sakurai, Nobuyoshi Miyajima, Hiroaki Ohfuji, Tomoo Katsura and Takafumi Yamamoto.
Science Advances, Vol. 3, no. 6, e1603024, DOI: 10.1126/sciadv.1603024, 07 Jun 2017.
http://advances.sciencemag.org/content/3/6/e1603024

Abstract

An open question for solid-Earth scientists is the amount of water in Earth's interior. The uppermost mantle and lower mantle contain little water because their dominant minerals, olivine and bridgmanite, have limited water storage capacity. In contrast, the mantle transition zone (MTZ) at a depth of 410 to 660 km is considered to be a potential water reservoir because its dominant minerals, wadsleyite and ringwoodite, can contain large amounts of water [up to 3 weight % (wt %)]. However, the actual amount of water in the MTZ is unknown. Given that water incorporated into mantle minerals can lower their viscosity, we evaluate the water content of the MTZ by measuring dislocation mobility, a property that is inversely proportional to viscosity, as a function of temperature and water content in ringwoodite and bridgmanite. We find that dislocation mobility in bridgmanite is faster by two orders of magnitude than in anhydrous ringwoodite but 1.5 orders of magnitude slower than in water-saturated ringwoodite. To fit the observed mantle viscosity profiles, ringwoodite in the MTZ should contain 1 to 2 wt % water. The MTZ should thus be nearly water-saturated globally.
++

CONCLUSION

THEORY # 4 EARTH'S DEEP MANTLE HAS THE WATER
FROM THE INTERSTELLAR MEDIUM

Researchers collected samples of primitive rocks from the Baffin Island, Nunavut Territory, Canada back in 1985. They analysed the samples and compared the Deuterium-to-Hydrogen Ratio (D/H Ratio) with that of seawater. The researchers found that the water contained in those primitive rocks of the Earth's deep mantle was the normal water, but not the heavy water (seawater). The Deuterium-to-Hydrogen Ratio (D/H Ratio) for sea water is known to be 1.56×10^{-4}. But researchers found that for the water collected from the primitive rock of deep mantle, the ratio was a lot less than 1.56×10^{-4}, indicating the fact that the water in the Earth's deep mantle is not deuterium-enriched, and so the water must have been inherited from the "interstellar medium", even before the formation of our Solar System, and survived in the deep mantle.

THEORY # 5 THICK HYDROGEN LAYER COULD HAVE REACTED WITH OXYGEN

V. RESEARCH FINDINGS ON WATER FORMATION
EARTH MADE ITS OWN WATER FROM A THICK HYDROGEN LAYER
THIS THEORY CHALLENGED ALL THE ABOVE-MENTIONED THEORIES
[162, 163]

Dr. Hidenori Genda and his colleague Dr. Masahiro Ikoma, from the Tokyo Institute of Technology, Tokyo, Japan suggest from their research study that the Earth had a thick atmosphere of hydrogen in the beginning, which reacted with oxides in the Earth's mantle to produce copious amounts of water.

Hydrogen could have reacted with oxygen available from the oxides of Earth's mantle, and could have formed water molecules. This water from the mantle could have been later transported to the Earth's surface, forming oceans. [$2 H_2 + O_2 = 2 H_2O$]

Thick Hydrogen Gas Layer: The evidence for the thick hydrogen shroud comes from the Earth's orbit. Its orbit, like those of Venus and Mars, is very circular now, but mathematical models suggest that it started out more elongated. If the planets were still submerged in a thick, hydrogen-rich solar nebula after they formed, however, the thick gas might have damped out any elongation of the orbits.

If the water on Earth did form from a thick hydrogen atmosphere, it should have originally had a far lower value of the deuterium-to-hydrogen ratio (D/H Ratio) than we see in oceans water today. The researchers argued, from relevant calculations, that the ratio would have naturally drifted upwards over time due the hydrogen layer depletion, loss of hydrogen from ocean's water, including the leakage of hydrogen into the space. Dr. Hidenori Genda and Dr. Masahiro Ikoma concluded from their calculations that the oceans might well have been chemically manufactured right here on Earth. The notion that Earth got its water by the bombardment of comets and/or asteroids (carbonaceous chondrites) could be false. They published a paper about their research finding as shown below.
+++

Journal Publication [163]

Origin of the Ocean on the Earth: Early Evolution of Water D/H in a Hydrogen-rich Atmosphere. Authors: Hidenori Genda, Masahiro Ikoma, Paper Submitted on 13 Sep 2007. Journal Reference: Icarus 194:42-52,2008.
https://arxiv.org/abs/0709.2025

Abstract

The origin of the Earth's ocean has been discussed on the basis of deuterium/hydrogen ratios (D/H) of several sources of water in the Solar System. The average D/H of carbonaceous chondrites (CC's) is known to be close to the current D/H of the Earth's ocean, while those of comets and the solar nebula are larger by about a factor of two and smaller by about a factor of seven, respectively, than that of the Earth's ocean. Thus, the main source of the Earth's ocean has been thought to be CC's or adequate mixing of comets and the solar nebula. However, those conclusions are correct only if D/H of water on the Earth has remained unchanged for the past 4.5 Gyr. In this paper, we investigate evolution of D/H in the ocean in the case that the early Earth had a hydrogen-rich atmosphere, the existence of which is predicted by recent theories of planet formation no matter whether the nebula remains or not. Then we show that D/H in the ocean increases by a factor of 2-9, which is caused by the mass fractionation during atmospheric hydrogen loss, followed by deuterium exchange between hydrogen gas and water vapor during ocean formation. This result suggests that the apparent similarity in D/H of water between CC's and the current Earth's ocean does not necessarily support the CC's origin of water and that the apparent discrepancy in D/H is not a good reason for excluding the nebular origin of water.

+++

CONCLUSION

THEORY # 5 THICK HYDROGEN LAYER COULD HAVE REACTED WITH OXYGEN
Another research paper suggested that hydrogen from the Earth's atmosphere could have reacted with oxygen available from the oxides of Earth's mantle, and could have formed water molecules in the mantle by the following chemical reaction [$2 H_2 + O_2 = 2 H_2O$].
This water from the mantle could have been later transported to the Earth's surface, forming oceans.

These researchers do not have supporting evidence with more research publications confirming that this is true. Moreover these researchers need to prove that the Earth did not inherit any water from the interstellar medium because there have been more research publications, confirming that the Earth inherited up to 50% of its water from the interstellar medium even before our Solar Sysyem was created.

+++

WATER FORMATION ON EARTH: YOUTUBE VIDEOS [164, 165, 166]

The following YouTube videos explain in simple language how our Earth possessed its water:

a. YouTube Title: Where did Earth's water come from? Narrated by Zachary Metz, TED-Ed Lessons, Published on Mar 23, 2015.
https://www.youtube.com/watch?v=RwtOo4EXgUE

SUMMARY: The theory of comets and asteroids brought water to Earth was refuted by some other scientists because of the following reason: Scientists analysed the samples of the rock from asteroids (Carbonaceous Chondrite or Meteorite). They found that D/H ratio and mineral composition of rocks of the Earth and of the Meteorites matched. Meteorite are originated from Asteroids. Therefore asteroids brought water to the Earth.

b. YouTube Title: Where Did Earth's Water Come From? by MinuteEarth, Published on Feb 7, 2014.
https://www.youtube.com/watch?v=_LpgBvEPozk

SUMMARY: Common sense tells that Earth could have gotten water from an external source such as comets, asteroids or meteorites such as carbonecious chondrites, which contain water as well as carbon. It was known to scientists that our planet Earth was bombarded by comets, asteroids and meteorites (such as carbonecious chondrites). If water came from the dirty ice-balls such as comets are logical candidates for the existence of water on Earth, but scientists found that the D/H ratio on comets is too high.

Comets are rich in heavy water (not the regular water).
So Earth's water could not have arrived from comets.

Water could have arrived from Carbonaceous Chondrite (a type of meteorite).
Carbonaceous Chondrite Meteorites contain a lot of water and carbon.

c. YouTube Title: How Did Earth Get Its Water? by SciShow Space, Published on May 31, 2016.
https://www.youtube.com/watch?v=_Y-XUAKTAkE

SUMMARY: Some water originally formed and stuck with the layers of Earth when it formed (Probably inherited from the interstellar medium). Some other water was brought by comets and asteroids.

+++

FINAL CONCLUSIONS: "THE ORIGIN OF THE EARTH'S WATER"
THE ORIGIN OF THE EARTH'S WATER REVEALED!

THEORIES OF WATER FORMATION ON OUR EARTH	CONCLUSION
1. COMETS COULD HAVE BROUGHT WATER TO EARTH • Our Solar System (Our Sun, Our Earth and other 7 Planets) began its formation 6 billion years ago, and completed its formation 4.54 billion years ago. Our ancestors believed that ice-bearing comets probably bombarded our Earth 4 to 3.8 billion years ago, and brought water to Earth. This theory is now believed to be wrong because (D/H Ratio) of the water from comets is much higher than that of ocean water. Our ancestors' belief that comets brought water to our planet Earth was however proved by our most recent scientists to be a myth.	MYTH!
2. ASTEROIDS (METEORITES /CARBONACEOUS CHONDRITES) COULD HAVE BROUGHT WATER TO EARTH • Water-rich asteroids (meteorites / carbonaceous chondrites) impacted the infant Earth about 4 to 3.8 billion years ago, distributing water across the planet by brute force. As a result, our oceans formed. This theory is more accurate because D/H Ratio of the water from asteroids matched well with that of ocean water. Research proved that our planet Earth attained up to 50% of its water from the asteroids during the early stages after the formation of our Solar System.	TRUE!
3. EARTH INHERITED ITS WATER FROM THE INTERSTELLAR MEDIUM • Water is known to form in the clouds of gas and dust of the interstellar medium (ISM). Our Solar System was created 6 billion years ago from a gigantic cloud of interstellar gas and stardust. That cloud collapsed and formed a solar nebula—a spinning, swirling disk of material under gravity. Scientists found that the primordial water of the interstellar medium survived within the particles of the stardust, and carried forward all the way until and after the formation our Earth. Researchers concluded, from an extensive experimental study and mathematical modelling, that our planet Earth inherited up to 50% of its water from the interstellar medium even before our Solar System was created. Our Solar System completed its formation 4.54 billion years ago. • However the water we drink today is at least 4.54 billion years old.	TRUE!
4. EARTH'S DEEP MANTLE HAS THE PRIMORDIAL WATER FROM THE INTERSTELLAR MEDIUM • The researchers collected samples of primitive rocks from the Baffin Island, Nunavut Territory, Canada back in 1985. Water analysis revealed that these rocks have lower amount of deuterium, and lower D/H Ratio, indicating that the Earth's deep mantle attained the primordial water from the interstellar medium. • Which means the water we drink today is at least 4.54 billion years old.	TRUE!
5. THICK HYDROGEN LAYER COULD HAVE REACTED WITH OXYGEN • Hydrogen could have reacted with oxygen available from the oxides of Earth's mantle, and could have formed water molecules after our Solar System formed. This water from the mantle could have been later transported to the Earth's surface, forming oceans. [$2 H_2 + O_2 = 2 H_2O$] • This theory does not have much supporting evidence and so disregarded.	FALSE!

FINAL CONCLUSIONS: "THE ORIGIN OF THE EARTH'S WATER"
THE ORIGIN OF THE EARTH'S WATER REVEALED!

◉ Astronomers, space researchers and scientists have known for decades that there is plenty of water in the interstellar medium. There is sufficient scientific research evidence along with journal publications supporting the fact that our planet Earth inherited primordial water from the interstellar medium even before our Solar System was created some 6 billion years ago.

◉ The water samples taken from our Earth's deep mantle (rocks found in 1985 from the Baffin Island, Nunavut Territory, Canada) were analysed and proved to contain primordial water formed in the interstellar medium. This discovery has given the strong supporting evidence that the water we drink today is at least 4.54 billion years old, older than our Solar System.

◉ Researchers compared the (D/H Ratio) of water samples taken from comets, asteroids (meteorites or carbonaceous chondrites), and concluded that the (D/H Ratio) of asteroids matched well with that of seawater, but did not match with that of comets (Oort cloud in the graph represents comets). The same researchers and several other researchers came to a conclusion that Earth's water did not come from comets, but perhaps up to 50% of water came from asteroids. However, there are some other scientists and researchers who still argue that Earth got its water neither from comets not from asteroids.

◉ A PhD thesis (of Ms. Ilsedore Cleeves, supervised by Dr. Edwin Ted Bergin, Professor and Chair in the Department of Astronomy, University of Michigan, Ann Arbor, Michigan, USA) was approved based on the scientific conclusion that <u>our planet Earth inherited up to 50% of its water from the interstellar medium, water was not completely evaporated after our Sun was born, but remained hidden within the dust particles until and after the formation of our planet Earth</u>. <u>Much of the water on our planet Earth and throughout our Solar System formation likely originated as ice deposited on the dust particles that formed in interstellar medium.</u> <u>The remaining 50% of the water might have resulted from the bombardment of asteroids (meteorites) during and after early stages of our Earth formation</u>. They published a paper about this discovery in the Science journal in 2014.

◉ **The intriguing idea** is that the ices from the interstellar medium were incorporated with a lot of organic material in them, which could have helped kick-start the life on our planet Earth.

How Did the Water Get Into The Interstellar Medium?

In order to form water in the interstellar medium, the following conditions must prevail:

(i) Both hydrogen and oxygen must abundantly be available under appropriate climate conditions (colder temperatures below -223 °C or 50 °K are necessary in most cases), and

(ii) The ionization of hydrogen molecules should readily be possible in order to take place the chemical reaction $2 H_2 + O_2 = 2 H_2O$.

◉ Nearly 380,000 years after the Big Bang, the primary element "hydrogen" was first created, and thereafter it was abundantly available throughout our Universe. Nearly 400 million years after the Big Bang, stars formation commenced using hydrogen as the burning fuel. The massive pressure build-up of the fiery inferno within the stars was so great that hydrogen atoms fused together to form heavier element helium.

Helium atoms in turn fused together to form much heavier elements such as lithium, beryllium, carbon, nitrogen, oxygen, and others in a process known as "**stellar nucleosynthesis**." The early stars were massive and short-lived. When the massive stars finished burning their hydrogen or helium fuel, they eventually extinguished, collapsed as they could not withstand their own gravitational force, and exploded into supernovae while manufacturing, dumping and scattering all kinds of heavier elements such as "carbon, nitrogen, oxygen, phosphorus and sulfur and many other elements" across the interstellar medium of our Milky Way Galaxy, and perhaps across the other galaxies our Universe.

🌑 More than 6 billion years ago, even before our Solar System and our Earth were created, during the supernova explosions in our Milky Way Galaxy, those newly formed heavier elements, including the very important oxygen, commingled together and formed all kinds of newer elements that we see in our periodic table today (there are 117 heavier elements).

🌑 Space scientists discovered that during the time when newer elements were being formed, the abundantly available hydrogen and oxygen commingled together in the star-forming clouds under the appropriate climate conditions, and formed ice-cold water molecules by the chemical reaction ($2 H_2 + O_2 = 2 H_2O$). Those ice-cold water molecules then entered into the space dust (also known as stardust) and interstellar gas in the interstellar medium, from a gigantic cloud of which our Solar System (our Sun, our planet Earth & 7 other planets) was created 6 billion years ago. The formation of our Solar System completed 4.54 billion years ago.

🌑 And that is how our planet Earth inherited liquid water even before it was born. Our planet Earth was thus born with water. The water we drink today is at least 4.54 billion years old, older than our planet Earth, older than our Sun, and older than our Solar System.

FORMATION OF LIFE ON OUR PLANET EARTH
LIFE FORMATION BASED ON
THE "WHOLE STORY FROM BIG BANG TO THE PRESENT DAY" [178, 179]

RECAP: If you could rewind your memory, our Universe was born 13.8 billion years ago. Some astronomers and scientists believe that first stars appeared after 200 million years, and others believe after 400 billion years. So the Milky Way began its formation 200 to 400 million years after the Big Bang. Therefore, our Milky Way Galaxy began its formation between 200 and 400 million years after the Big Bang, which means our Milky Way Galaxy is approximately 13.4 billion years to 13.6 years old. The spiral-shaped Milky Way Galaxy is one of the 2 trillion galaxies in our mysterious Universe upon which we all live. Our Solar System (our Sun, our planet Earth, our Moon and 7 other planets) is located on Milky Way Galaxy on one of the spiral arms, and began its formation 6 billion years ago, and completed its formation 4.54 billion years ago. The age of our planet Earth, our Sun and our Solar System was determined by radiometric dating (which is the most accurate and reliable method to date old rocks) as 4.54 billion years.

Over the next 8.6 billion years (**Until 4.6 Billion Years Ago**), the explosions of supernovas continued, stars exploded, and reborn over and over again. Obviously, the Milky Way Galaxy has been thereby filled with a variety of stardust clouds occurred during the explosions and star formations.

About 4.4 Billion Years Ago: It was too hot on Earth for liquid water to exist. Water evaporated and steam generated into the atmosphere. For millions of years, as the planet cools, rain pours down, forming ponds, lakes, rivers and eventually our oceans.

About 3.8 Billion Years Ago: About 3.8 billion years ago, our planet Earth had water, oceans and Moon. But oxygen was not yet available on Earth for the life to exist. 700,000 years after the planet Earth first formed, life on Earth emerged. Tiny organisms such as bacteria started growing on the bottom surface of the oceans. Bacteria is the most important life formation organism. In fact, all our bodies still possess tons of bacteria living in our bodies, without which survival is not possible. For billions of years, microbes grew in the oceans and spread all over the oceans.

About 2.5 Billion Years Ago: About 2.5 billion years ago, some kind of bacteria, more specifically cyanobacteria, figured out the clue on how to consume Sunshine and produce waste product such as "oxygen" by photosynthesis. The ocean floor was then filled with oxygen. The iron particles in the ocean floor combined with oxygen, and produced red-colored iron oxide (rusted iron). These iron deposits on the ocean floor drove the industrial revolution in the later part of humanity. The bacteria produced vast amounts of oxygen in the oceans, and released into the Earth's atmosphere. Some organisms started living by breathing oxygen. But after sometime, all the iron was used up in the ocean floor, and then the bacteria started ejecting the excess oxygen into the atmosphere. So the atmosphere has the oxygen by now. This period, 2.3 billion years ago, marks the start of the Great Oxygenation Event (GOE), which was followed by further increases later in Earth's history.

About 2.5 Billion Years Ago: Over the next 2 billion years, the Earth passed through many complex transformations and changes. The sky became blue, plants grew and Earth has become a stable place, filled with oxygen, nitrogen, carbon, and all other elements of our periodic table.

FORMATION OF THE OXYGEN ON OUR PLANET EARTH

About 550 Million Years Ago: Our planet Earth is now 4.54 billion years old. It took 4 billion years for the Earth to become an inhabitable place in our Universe. Oxygen levels in the Earth's atmosphere have risen to 13%. The current oxygen level in the atmosphere is 21%.

• For the first 50 million years, all kinds of strange creatures were born in the ocean floor and on the surface of Earth. About 500 million years ago, the first bony fish was born in the ocean. These fish were our direct ancestors. Those fish represented the models of human beings by possessing the bony spine, head with teeth, nose, eyes and ears.

• For the first 50 million years, the bacteria and plants grew inside the oceans. But that is all going to change (from microbes to humans) during the next 500 million years.

• During the next few million years, ozone layer (O_3) around the Earth's atmosphere was created from oxygen in order to protect us from Sun's radiations.

About 400 Million Years Ago: About 400 million years ago, the animals were born. The first generation of animals appeared on the planet Earth were amphibians. Amphibians are cold-blooded, which means that they had the same temperature as the air or water around them. There are more than 4,000 different kinds of amphibians. Members of this animal class are frogs, toads, salamanders, newts, and caecilians or blindworms. They evolved to generate a new form of eggs with the shell that keeps the moisture so that the eggs would have life in them. Even if the eggs are far away from water, they survive with the moisture of the eggs. That is the way humans were able to colonize the rest of the land for life to spread, even without water. Then the next generation of the animals were reptiles.

About 300 Million Years Ago: About 300 million years ago, many types of plants grew on the surface of Earth, but were dead and buried underground due the high heat produced by the Sun.

About 250 Million Years Ago: About 250 million years ago, a kind of apocalypse evolved. Volcanic activity took over the planet Earth. The atmosphere was filled with carbon dioxide (CO_2). More than 70% of all the species on Earth went extinct. It was the very massive extinction. Up to this point in time, extinction took place more than half a dozen times, and new creatures took over the planet.

About 250 Million Years Ago: About 250 million years ago, a kind of apocalypse evolved. Volcanic activity took over the planet Earth. The atmosphere was filled with carbon dioxide (CO_2). More than 70% of all the species on Earth went extinct. It was the very massive extinction. Up to this point in time, extinction took place more than half a dozen times, and new creatures took over the planet.

65 Million Years Ago Dinosours Lived: At the time of dinosaurs, an asteroid (a 6-mile wide object) strikes the Earth. Dust cloud blocked the Sun, and as a result the temperatures plummeted rapidly. The dinosaurs were all dead, and the era of dinosaurs was over. After that, the mammals were born with five fingers similar to humans.

50 Million Years Ago: Our ancestors began the life. Scientists examined the Egyptian pyramids today, and determined that some of those pyramids were made with 50 million year old seashells, made of limestone.

10 Million Years Ago: The Earth was transformed into more mature planet than ever, comforting the life formation. Many rivers formed. Mountains like Himalayans rose.

7 Million Years Ago: The grasslands showed up with trees and forests, all around the planet Earth. Some creatures lived on trees. Apes (our ancestors) were born and started living on the trees.

2.6 Million Years Ago Early Humanoids Lived: Early, having an appearance or character resembling that of a human, appeared on the planet Earth. They started creating and using silicon stones such as hammer-like tools and cutting tools to break the rocks and started using them to build walls. Silicon launches the very first technological revolution called the stone-age.

800,000 years ago: Our ancestors learned to generate fire, as the fire was easy to made from forest trees and plenty of oxygen available on Earth's atmosphere. Fire was the cause of internal combustion engine. Fire has become the source of energy for the humans to move forward. Humans have become intelligent beings and learned to convert clay into pottery, metals into weaponry, and water into steam. They learned to cook foods using fire.

200,000 Years Ago: Modern humans have emerged on to the planet Earth, and began to speak and communicate. As a species, humans have become exponentially smarter and intelligent beings. They began to speak, sharing information and communicating each other.

100,000 Years Ago: Humans started moving with primitive tools, walking, eating, drinking and communicating in the ancient African continent. Migrating to other continents for better life has become a hobby.

50,000 Years ago: Glaciers began to emerge. Ice-age has began.

30,000 Years Ago: Homo Sapiens (In Latin: "Homo Sapien=Wise Man") reached Europe from Africa for the first time. Homo sapiens, the species to which all modern human beings belong. Homo sapiens is one of several species grouped into the genus Homo, but it is the only one that is not extinct.

20,000 Years Ago: Humans have advanced to become intellectual beings, and began to easily adapt to cold atmosphere by using shelters and clothing.

12,000 to 5,000 Years Ago:
* By 10,000 BC, people started migrating from Africa to South Amerca, and then the entire globe. People started adapting to cold climate, and started civilizing. Sea levels rose again, and humans were separated by continents. As glaciers spread, the lakes and rivers generated. These rivers and valleys allowed humans to form the first seeds of civilization.
* After the ice-age, temperatures rose, our planet warmed up, plants grew with all kinds of vegetation, and all kinds of animals grew with emerging population.
* Humans migrated from Siberia to North America. Migration for a better life has became a hobby.
* Humans learned to plant seeds, and cultivate agriculture so that the increased population would have enough food (grains, vegetables, greens, fruits, spices, nuts & seeds) to consume.
* Then the human population grew tremendously, and thereafter we have recorded evidence of all kinds of human activities that took place on our planet Earth.

RECORDED EVIDENCE OF HUMAN EVOLUTION [180]

Charles Darwin (1809–1882) published a revolutionary book in 1859 titled "On the Origin of Species by Means of Natural Selection." Darwin insisted that all living things, including humans, achieved their present form through a long period of evolution process. But Darwin's theorem did not include documented scientific evidence that apes are indeed evolved to become humans. However nobody really knew, and nobody witnessed if apes were indeed transformed into human bodies. Especially human brain is no match to ape's brain.

The following evidence was gathered from recorded historical facts by anthropologists:
The following terminology is necessary to understand the human evolution:
Paleontologists study fossils (fossils are bones and teeth from human remains).
Anthropologists study humans and their origins, development, and customs.
Anatomists study the structure of biological organisms in the living things.
Biochemists study chemical processes occurring in biological organisms.
Scientists study the circumstances based on science and laws of physics.
Fossils: Remains or imprints of ancient plants or animals that are found in layers of rock.
Hominid: Member of the family of primates that includes modern humans.
Primate: Member of the group of mammals that includes lemurs, monkeys, apes, and humans.

There is no recorded evidence that human life began before 4.4 million years ago (Our Earth is 4.54 billion years old). However, a species named "Australopithecus Afarensis" lived 3.18 million years ago.

Australopithecus (nicknamed Lucy) Lived 3.18 Million Years Ago: These are one of the oldest known humanlike animals. On November 24, 1974, at the site of Hadar in Ethiopia, a team of anthropologists led by an American paleoanthropologist named Donald Johanson (1943) documented that Australopithecus (nicknamed Lucy) lived about 3.18 million years ago. Lucy was only 3 feet 8 inches (1.1 m) tall, weighed 29 kilograms (65 lb) and looked somewhat like a Common Chimpanzee, but the observations of her pelvis proved that: Lucy had walked upright and more in the manner of humans. Lucy had a skull, knees, and a pelvis more similar to humans than to apes. In 1924, Australian anthropologist Raymond Dart (1893–1988) discovered fossils at a site called Taung in South Africa. These fossils, dated at 3 million years old, were named Australopithecus africanus, meaning the southern ape of Africa.

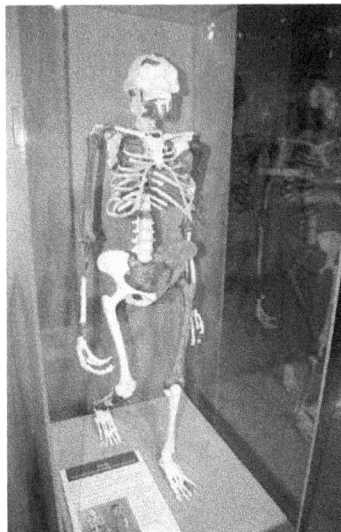

Figure 20.6 Lucy skeleton reconstruction at the Cleveland (OHIO, USA) Museum of Natural History. [181]

Homo Sapiens Appeared 400,000 Years Ago: Between 250,000 and 400,000 years ago, Homo erectus evolved into Homo sapiens. It is interesting to note here that these ancestors of modern man cooked their food, wore clothing, buried their dead, and constructed shelters, but did not have a modern-sized brain. Over time, the body and brain of Homo sapiens gradually became somewhat larger.

Cro-Magnon Appeared 40,000 Years Ago: By about 40,000 years ago, Homo sapiens had evolved into modern human beings. Homo sapien, in Latin, means Wise Man. In 1868, the first fossils of modern Homo sapiens were found in Cro-Magnon caves in southwest France, which gave that name to all early Homo sapiens. Cro-Magnon remains have been found along with the skeletons of woolly mammoth, bison, and reindeer and with tools made from bone, antler, ivory, stone, and wood, indicating that Cro-Magnon hunted game of all sizes. Cro-Magnon also buried their dead relatives with body ornaments such as necklaces, beaded clothing, and bracelets.

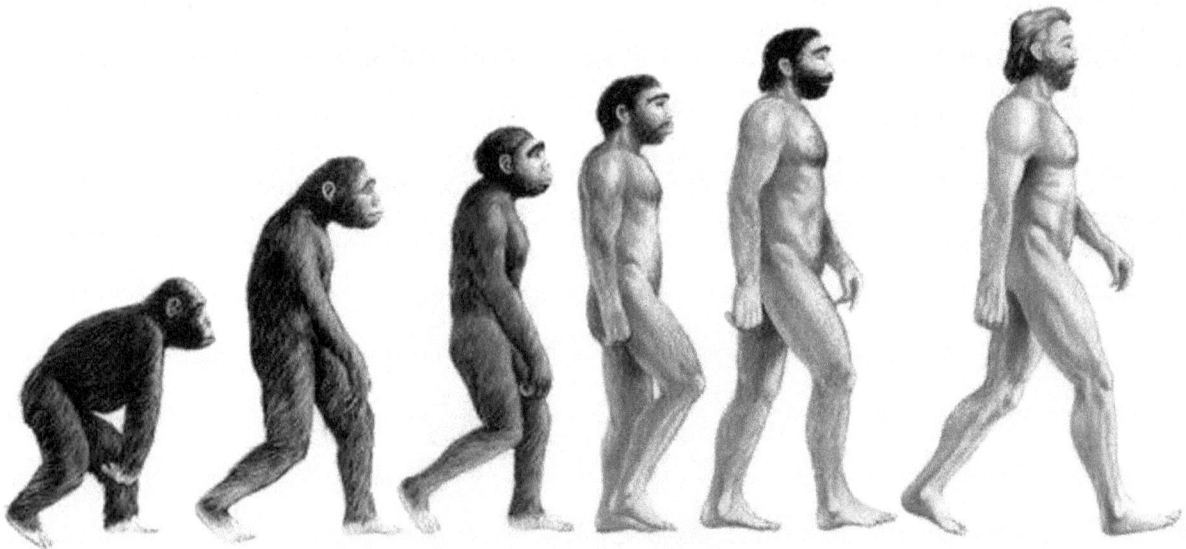

Neanderthals Lived Until 35,000 Years Ago and Then Disappeared:
Neanderthals appeared some 300,000 years ago in Europe, lived throughout the ice ages, and disappeared about 35,000 years ago. These humanlike hominids lived in caves and had a large brain, a strong upper body, a bulbous nose, and a prominent brow ridge. They were proficient hunters. It is possible that Neanderthals had an elaborate culture, and were aware of the medicinal properties of plants. They also ritually buried their dead relatives with body ornaments such as necklaces, beaded clothing, and bracelets.

Figure 20.7 Theory of Evolution from Ape to Homo Sapien.

SEVEN THEORIES ON THE ORIGIN OF LIFE
POSTED BY CHARLES Q. CHOI, LIVE SCIENCE CONTRIBUTOR [182]

Based on the scientific evidence available to astronomers and scientists, the following seven theories are being derived and proposed with regards to the origin of life formation on the planet Earth:

It is known to astronomers and scientists that the Earth was born 4.54 billion years ago. Life on Earth began more than 3 billion years ago from the primordial soup, evolved from the most basic of microbes into a dazzling array of complex organisms over time. Primordial soup is a liquid substance that existed on Earth before there were any plants, animals, or humans and from which plants, animals, and humans developed.

Theory # 1: Life Kick-Started With An Electric Spark
Lightning may have provided the spark needed for life to begin. It is known to scientists that an electric spark can generate amino acids and sugars from an atmosphere loaded with water, methane, ammonia and hydrogen, as was shown in the famous Miller-Urey experiment reported in 1953. This experiment suggests that lightning might have helped kick-start and create the key building blocks of life on Earth in its early days. Over millions of years, smaller molecules were evolved into larger and more complex molecules.

Theory # 2: Molecules of Life Met on Clay
The first molecules of life might have met on clay, according to an idea elaborated by organic chemist Alexander Graham Cairns-Smith at the University of Glasgow in Scotland. These clay surfaces might have been concentrated and clogged together with the pertinent organic compounds, and helped organize them into patterns much like our genes do now. The main role of DNA is to store information on how other molecules should be arranged. Genetic sequences in DNA are essentially instructions on how amino acids should be arranged in proteins. Cairns-Smith suggested that mineral crystals in clay could have arranged organic molecules into organized patterns. After a while, organic molecules took over this job and organized themselves to form more complex life-bearing organisms.

Theory # 3: Life Began Under Deep-Sea Vents
The deep-sea vent theory suggests that life may have begun at submarine hydrothermal vents spewing key hydrogen-rich molecules. Their rocky nooks could then have concentrated these molecules together and provided mineral catalysts for critical reactions to take place. Those vents, rich in chemical and thermal energy, sustained vibrant ecosystems. The necessary critical reactions continued within the deep-dea vents until the basic microbes formed from which more complex organisms developed.

Theory # 4: Life Had a Chilly Start
It is believed that around 3 billion years ago, our oceans were covered by a thick layer of ice, possibly hundreds of feet thick. The Sun at that time was about 3 times less luminous and less intense than it is now. This thick layer of ice probably contained the fragile organic matter and the relevant chemical compounds necessary to form life. This thick layer of ice protected the life formation underneath from the dangerous ultraviolet radiation from the Sun and from the destruction that might have caused by cosmic rays impacts. The cold temperatures underneath the thick layer of ice might have also helped these organic molecules to grow and survive longer periods, allowing key reactions to occur for the life formation.

Theory # 5: The Answer Lies in Understanding DNA Formation

DNA = Deoxyribo Nucleic Acid
RNA = Ribo Nucleic Acid
PNA = Peptide Nucleic Acid
TNA = Threose Nucleic Acid
Deoxyribo Nucleic Acid (DNA) is a self-replicating material present in nearly all living organisms as the main constituent of chromosomes. Chromosome is a thread-like structure of nucleic acids and protein found in the nucleus of most living cells, carrying genetic information used in the growth, development, functioning and reproduction of all known living organisms and many viruses in the form of genes. It is the carrier of genetic information.

It is known to scientists that the formation of DNA needs proteins, and on the other hand the formation of proteins need DNA. This dilemma has been resolved by understanding RNA. RNA stores information similar to DNA, also serves as enzyme-like proteins, and helps create both DNA and proteins. Once the DNA was formed from RNA, both DNA and proteins overtook the process because they are more efficient in their functions. Scientists have also discovered the other nucleic acids such as PNA and TNA, which may have given birth to the formation of RNA. However it is still unknown if either one of these molecules could have spontaneously arisen on to the planet Earth from the gas and dust of the interstellar medium, which coalesced over millions of years during the formation the planet Earth. The scientists still have find out the origin of the DNA to make sure whether the Earth originally possessed the DNA molecules or they have been implanted later by the space objects during the development of Earth's atmosphere.

Theory # 6: Life Had Simple Beginnings
Instead of developing from complex molecules such as RNA, life might have begun with smaller molecules interacting with each other in cycles of reactions. These might have been contained in simple capsules akin to cell membranes, and over time more complex molecules that performed these reactions better than the smaller ones could have evolved, scenarios dubbed "metabolism-first" models, as opposed to the "gene-first" model of the "RNA world" hypothesis.

Theory # 7: Research Showed that Life Was Brought Here from Elsewhere!
Life Hitchhiked At First to Comets, Asteroids or Meteorites, and Then to Our Planet Earth!
Panspermia: Life did not begin on Earth at all, but was brought here from elsewhere in space, a notion known as "panspermia." Panspermia theory states that life was first created in the Universe at one spot, and then spread throughout the Universe, from planet to planet and then from galaxy to galaxy. Panspermia is a theory that states that life on our Earth originated from microorganisms or chemical precursors of life present in outer space and able to initiate life upon reaching a suitable environment. For instance, rocks regularly get blasted off our neighboring planet Mars by cosmic impacts, and it is true a number of Martian meteorites have been found on our Earth.

Microorganisms were carefully trapped inside the rocky material of comets, asteroids and/or meteorites. That rocky material was wrapped by an icy layer to protect it from damage or destruction of microorganisms. That icy layer was further covered by clay or spacedust. The spacedust shielded and protected the microorganisms from ultraviolet (UV) radiations transmitted from the Sun. Thus the microorganisms were safely transported to our planet Earth from elsewhere in the space in order for the life to initiate and propagate. Those microorganisms then grew up into complex formations of life, including the formation and growth of humans. "In other words, life might have hitchhiked at first to comets, asteroids and/or meteorites during their bombardment, and then to our planet Earth from the other solar systems of our Milky Way Galaxy, or even from the other galaxies of our Universe."

ARE WE ALL REALLY MADE OF STARDUST?

NASA's scientists, astronomers and space researchers studied extensively the possibility of the formation and existence of life in the other planets of our Solar System, and always adopted that "Life requires 6 essential elements to survive such as CHNOPS: carbon, hydrogen, nitrogen, oxygen, phosphorus and sulfur." All organisms are built from the same 6 elements.

Scientists also believe that all the elements such as oxygen, carbon, hydrogen and nitrogen, sodium, calcium, magnesium, iron, zinc, copper, selenium, chromium, manganese, and many other trace minerals that are needed for human body formation and survival, and many other heavier elements such as iron, steel, copper that are needed for our houses, buildings and bridges were inherited by our planet Earth from the stardust generated by supernova explosions.

All those elements of our periodic table, shown below, were believed to be present in the stardust produced from supernova explosions. A dominant portion of our physical bodies are made out of stardust as it contains all the elements that a physical human body needs.

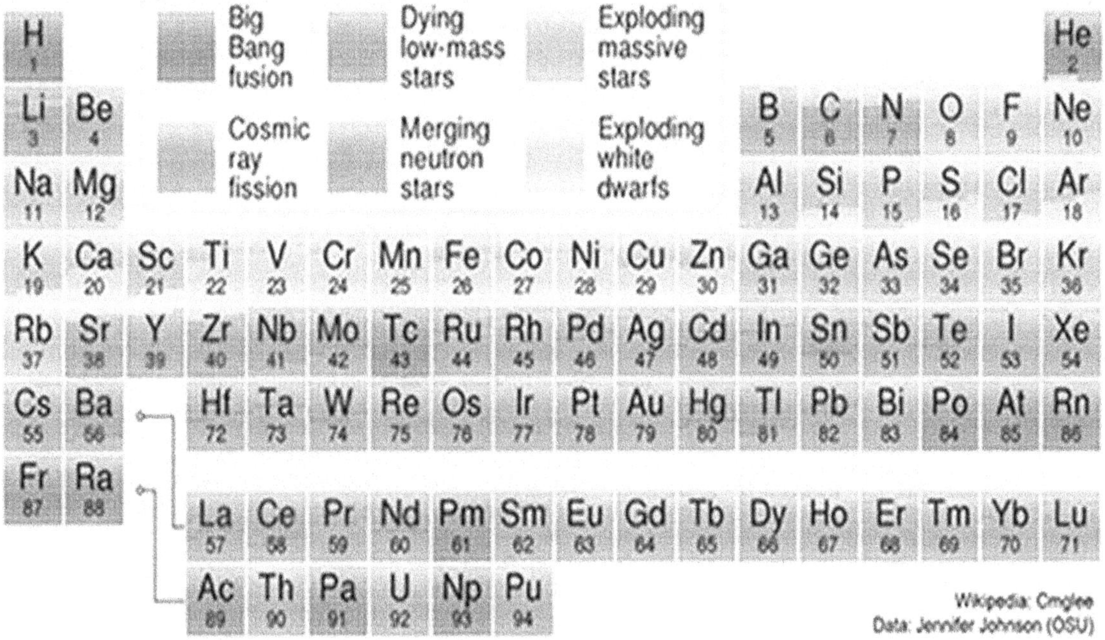

Figure 20.5 Periodic Table (All these elements were created in stars & scattered by supernovae).

This may sound unbelievable, but the scientific truth is that almost every element found on Earth was created in the burning core of collapsing stars, all the stuff that makes up life on Earth, including our bodies are made from stardust (at least 90%). NASA's scientists have studied stardust extensively, and came up with the aforementioned conclusion. [183]

NASA Posted: The hydrogen in your body, present in every molecule of water, came from the Big Bang. There are no other appreciable sources of hydrogen in our Universe. The carbon in your body was made by nuclear fusion in the interior of stars, as was the oxygen. Much of the iron in your body was made during supernovas of stars that occurred long ago and far away. The gold in your jewelry was likely made from neutron stars during collisions that may have been visible as short-duration gamma-ray bursts or gravitational wave events. Elements like phosphorus and copper are present in our bodies in only small amounts but are essential to the functioning of all known life. [184]

Astronomer Dr. Carl Sagan Wrote In His Book "Cosmos" The Following: [185]
"The nitrogen in our DNA, the calcium in our teeth, the iron in our blood, the carbon in our apple pies were made in the interiors of collapsing stars (which explode into supernovae). We are all made of starstuff."

Carl Pettit Also Posted the Following: [186]
Human beings are literally made out of star stuff. Almost all of the chemical elements (except hydrogen) that make up a person came from the stars. Any element heavier than hydrogen originated in the stars, and we are definitely composed of more than hydrogen. Calcium, carbon, hydrogen, nitrogen, oxygen and around 60 other basic ingredients make up a human being. Since hydrogen and helium were the only elements around before the stars manufactured in their burning cores, it's a safe bet that most of the substances that constitutes the "physical you" came from the stars.

The Wilkinson Microwave Anisotropy Probe (WMAP) determined that about 4.6% of the mass and energy of our Universe is contained in atoms (protons and neutrons). All of life is made from a portion of this 4.6%. The only chemical elements created at the beginning of our Universe were hydrogen, helium and lithium, which are the three lightest atoms in the periodic table. These elements were formed throughout our Universe as a hot gas. If you imagine a Universe where elements heavier than lithium would never form, then in that case life would never develop. But that is not what happened in our Universe. We are carbon-based life forms but not hydrogen-based life forms. We are made up of water and we drink water as more than 60% of the adult bodies are water. We breathe oxygen. Carbon and oxygen were not created in the Big Bang, but rather much later in stars. All of the carbon and oxygen in all living things are made in the nuclear fusion reactors that we call stars. The early stars were massive and short-lived. They consume their own hydrogen, helium and lithium and produce much heavier elements when they die. When these stars die and explode into supernovae, they dump and spread the elements of life, such as carbon and oxygen, throughout the interstellar medium of our Universe. Supernova explosions give birth to new Solar Systems along with orbiting planets that are enriched with all kinds of heavier elements that we see in our periodic table today. The stage is set for life to begin. Understanding when and how these events occur offer another window on the evolution of life, not only in our galaxy but also in other galaxies of our Universe. [187]

Almost 99% of the mass of the human body is made up SIX essential elements "carbon, hydrogen, nitrogen, oxygen, phosphorus and sulfur (CHNOPS)." Only about 0.85% is composed of another five elements: potassium, sulfur, sodium, chlorine, and magnesium. All 11 elements are necessary for the formation and survival of life. The remaining elements are in trace amounts. [188]

About 96 percent of the mass of the human body is made up of just four elements: oxygen, carbon, hydrogen and nitrogen, with a lot of that in the form of water, and the remaining 4% of the body mass is made up of all the other elements shown in our periodic table (there are 177 elements except hydrogen) in trace amounts. [189]

The FDA (Food and Drug Administration) of USA has set a minimum standard for the daily intake of 12 minerals such as calcium, iron, phosphorous, iodine, magnesium, zinc, selenium, copper, manganese, chromium, molybdenum and chloride. In addition, silicon, boron, nickel, vanadium and lead play an important role in biological formulations within our bodies. [189]

Approximately oxygen (65%) and hydrogen (10%) are predominantly found in water, which makes up about 60 percent of an adult body weight. It's practically impossible to imagine life on Earth or in any other planet without water. [189]

Human beings are a carbon-based life form. Carbon (18%) is synonymous with life. Its central role is due to the fact that it has four bonding sites that allow for the building of long, complex chains of molecules. Carbon atoms make up an immense part of our bodies molecular structure. Carbon is an essential component of the human diet. Luckily, carbon is easily and abundantly available in foods such as vegetables, fruits, grains, and meats. [189]

Another important element for the human body survival is nitrogen, which is obtained from the nitrates present in drinking water, and also from vegetables, fruits, dairy products, fish and meats. In addition, trace amounts of sodium, calcium, magnesium, iron, zinc, copper, selenium, chromium, manganese, molybdenum, cobalt, phosphorus, potassium, sulphur, chlorine, fluorine, iodine, and all the remaining elements of the periodic table are essential for the human body survival. [189]

Healthy Eating Habits Are Therefore Necessary:

⊕ Our bodies get all the aforementioned trace elements by consuming a balanced meal every single day. Stop eating all those greasy foods in restaurants. Eat at home well-balanced meals throughout the day. Make sure that every meal you consume (either small meal or big meal), there is some protein in it. Consume whole foods only, and avoid processed foods and refined foods. Consume well-balanced meals with oven-baked skinless & boneless chicken, turkey or fish, a variety of organic vegetables and dark-leafy greens, legumes, a variety of organic fruits, grains, nuts and seeds so that your body would get sufficient amount of protein, fat and carbs, all kinds of vitamins, minerals and fiber. Please maintain high self-discipline to strictly avoid processed meat products. Consume plenty of organic egg whites (discard the yolk) daily to boost your protein consumption. Did you know egg-white is one 100% protein and one 100% safe?

Healthy Water-Drinking Habits Are Therefore Extremely Important:
Make Your Own Nutritious Mineral Water from Purified Water at Home:

⊕ Please do not drink tap water, well water, or bottled water of any kind without knowing how pure it is. Please always drink purified water (RO water, distilled water, or zero water). And learn how to remineralize and alkalize the purified water at home.

⊕ Purified water that is either neutralized (pH=7) or slightly alkalized (pH=7 to 7.25), and remineralizedup up to a TDS (Total Dissolved Solids) level of 200 ppm is the healthy drinking water! Please refer to Drinking Water Guide (Chapter 14, Chapter 17, Chapter 18 & Chapter 19) and learn how to make and drink that kind of water.

⊕ There are more than 10 experiments conducted at home in Chapter 14, Chapter 17 & Chapter 18 of the complete book "Drinking Water Guide." Any reasonable person with minimal scientific background would be able to read and understand these experiments, and would be able to make his/her nutritious mineral water at home. This is the clean and healthy water you must drink at least 8 cups a day.

REFERENCES
There are no references from 1 to 79. This chapter begins with Reference number 80.

WATER FORMATION
80. Oceans Worlds, Water in the Solar System and Beyond by NASA.
https://www.nasa.gov/specials/ocean-worlds/

81. Water, water, everywhere in our Solar system but what does that mean for life? Posted on April 20, 2017.
https://theconversation.com/water-water-everywhere-in-our-solar-system-but-what-does-that-mean-for-life-76315

82. Origin of water in the solar system is interstellar by Michael Küffmeier, Daily Paper Summarie, Posted on Dec 9, 2014.
https://astrobites.org/2014/12/09/origin-of-water-in-the-solar-system-is-interstellar/

83. Deuterium, from Wikipedia.
https://en.wikipedia.org/wiki/Deuterium

84. Difference Between Heavy Water and Normal Water by Madhusha, Posted on August 1, 2017.
http://pediaa.com/difference-between-heavy-water-and-normal-water/

85. The First Three Minutes, Astronomy 162 by Professor Barbara Ryden.
http://www.astronomy.ohio-state.edu/~ryden/ast162_10/notes44.html

86. Primordial Nucleosynthesis and the Abundances of the Light Elements by Astro 2201.
http://www.astro.cornell.edu/academics/courses/astro201/primordnuc.htm

87. What is Deuterium? by Qlarivia.
https://qlarivia.com/what-is-deuterium/

88. Deuterium in Nature by Qlarivia.
https://qlarivia.com/about-deuterium/deuterium-in-water/

89. Asteroids Battered Young Earth Longer Than Thought by Charles Q. Choi, Space.com Contributor, Posted on April 25, 2012.
https://www.space.com/15424-asteroids-battered-Earth-collisions.html

90. The Late Heavy Bombardment Ends by BBC, UK.
http://www.bbc.co.uk/science/Earth/Earth_timeline/late_heavy_bombardment

COMETS COULD HAVE BROUGHT WATER TO EARTH
91. Did comets bring water to Earth? by Kimberly M. Burtnyk, Space, Posted on June 13, 2012.
http://Earthsky.org/space/did-comets-bring-water-to-Earth

92. Journal Publication: Ocean-like water in the Jupiter-family comet 103P/Hartley 2. Authors: Paul Hartogh, Dariusz C. Lis, Dominique Bockelée-Morvan, Miguel de Val-Borro, Nicolas Biver, Michael Küppers, Martin Emprechtinger, Edwin A. Bergin, Jacques Crovisier, Miriam Rengel, Raphael Moreno, Slawomira Szutowicz & Geoffrey A. Blake, Nature, Volume 478, pages 218–220 (13 October 2011).
https://www.nature.com/articles/nature10519

93. Rosetta Spacecraft: To Catch a Comet by Tim Sharp, Reference Editor, Posted on February 27, 2017.
https://www.space.com/24292-rosetta-spacecraft.html

94. Water On Rosetta's Comet Different To Water On Earth by IFL Science.
http://www.iflscience.com/space/rosetta-data-suggests-water-Earth-probably-didnt-come-comets/

95. Rosetta Results: Comets 'did not bring water to Earth' by Rebecca Morelle, Science Correspondent, BBC News, Posted on December 10, 2014.
https://www.bbc.com/news/science-environment-30414519

96. Most of Earth's Water Came from Asteroids, Not Comets by Charles Q. Choi, Space.com Contributor, Posted on December 10, 2014.
https://www.space.com/27969-Earth-water-from-asteroids-not-comets.html

97. Rosetta fuels debate on origin of Earth's oceans, Posted on December 10, 2014.
http://sci.esa.int/rosetta/55116-rosetta-fuels-debate-on-origin-of-Earths-oceans/

98. Journal Publication: Rosetta Mission
67P/Churyumov-Gerasimenko, a Jupiter family comet with a high D/H ratio
Authors: K. Altwegg1,*, H. Balsiger1, A. Bar-Nun2, J. J. Berthelier3, A. Bieler1,4, P. Bochsler1, C. Briois5, U. Calmonte1, M. Combi4, Science Vol. 347, Issue 6220, 1261952, Jan 23, 2015.
http://science.sciencemag.org/content/347/6220/1261952

ASTEROIDS COULD HAVE BROUGHT WATER TO EARTH

99. How Did Water Come to Earth? by Brian Greene, Smithsonian Magazine, Posted in May 2013.
https://www.smithsonianmag.com/science-nature/how-did-water-come-to-Earth-72037248/

100. Where did Earth's (and the asteroid belt's) water come from? by Sean Raymond, Posted on July 5, 2017.
https://planetplanet.net/2017/07/05/inner-solar-system-water/

101. Primitive Meteorites Brought Water To Early Earth by IFL Science.
http://www.iflscience.com/space/primitive-meteorites-brought-water-early-Earth/

102. Was Earth All Land Before? Scientists Unravel the Mystery by Alfred Kristoffer A. Guiang, Posted on Oct 31, 2014.
http://www.sciencetimes.com/articles/1116/20141031/Earth-land-before-scientists-unravel-mystery.htm

103. Mystery of Earth's water origin finally solved? It may be older than you think by Rhodi Lee, Tech Times, Posted on October 31, 2014.
https://www.techtimes.com/articles/19151/20141031/mystery-of-earths-water-origin-finally-solved-it-may-be-older-than-you-think.htm

104. Meteorites Brought Water To Earth During the First Two Million Years by Elizabeth Howell, Posted on Jan 18, 2018.
https://www.astrobio.net/news-exclusive/meteorites-brought-water-to-Earth-during-the-first-two-million-years/

105. Meteorites Brought Water To Earth During the First Two Million Years of Our Solar System, Astrobiology at NASA, Life in the Universe.
https://astrobiology.nasa.gov/news/meteorites-brought-water-to-Earth-during-the-first-two-million-years/

106. Mystery of Earth's Water Origin Solved by Andrew Fazekas, For National Geographic, Posted on October 30, 2014.
https://news.nationalgeographic.com/news/2014/10/141030-starstruck-Earth-water-origin-vesta-science/

107. New Study Finds Oceans Arrived Early to Earth by Woods Hole Oceanographic Institution, Posted on October 13, 2014.
https://www.whoi.edu/news-release/OriginEarthWater

108. New study finds oceans arrived early to Earth, Woods Hole Oceanographic Institution, Posted on October 30, 2014.
https://phys.org/news/2014-10-oceans-early-Earth.html

109. Journal Publication
Early accretion of water in the inner solar system from a carbonaceous chondrite–like source. Authors: Adam R. Sarafian, Sune G. Nielsen, Horst R. Marschall, Francis M. McCubbin, Brian D. Monteleone, Science, Vol. 346, Issue 6209, pp. 623-626, 31 Oct 2014.
http://science.sciencemag.org/content/346/6209/623

110. Carbonaceous Chondrites as Source of Earth's Water by Enrico de Lazaro, Posted on Jul 16, 2012.
http://www.sci-news.com/space/article00466.html

111. Water, Carbonaceous Chondrites, and Earth by CosmoSparks.
http://www.psrd.hawaii.edu/CosmoSparks/July12/Earthwater-sources.html

112. Journal Publication
The Provenances of Asteroids, and Their Contributions to the Volatile Inventories of the Terrestrial Planets, Authors: C. M. O'D. Alexander, R. Bowden, M. L. Fogel, K. T. Howard, C. D. K. Herd, L. R. Nittler, Science, Vol. 337, Issue 6095, pp. 721-723, DOI: 10.1126/ Science.1223474, Aug 10, 2012.
http://science.sciencemag.org/content/337/6095/721.full?sid=aa2da622-520a-4813-b0b5-30bdc95f33bf

113. Earth's Water Likely Came from Very Early Asteroid Strikes by Mike Wall, Senior Writer, LiveScience, Posted on October 25, 2013.
https://www.livescience.com/40699-Earth-water-origin-asteroid-impacts.html

114. Journal Publication
Vortex magnetic structure in framboidal magnetite reveals existence of water droplets in an ancient asteroid. Authors: Yuki Kimura, Takeshi Sato, Norihiro Nakamura, Jun Nozawa, Tomoki Nakamura, Katsuo Tsukamoto & Kazuo Yamamoto Nature Communications volume 4, Article number: 2649, October 22, 2013.
https://www.nature.com/articles/ncomms3649

115. Journal Publication
A dual origin for water in carbonaceous asteroids revealed by CM chondrites.
Authors: Laurette Piani, Hisayoshi Yurimoto & Laurent Remusat
Nature Astronomy, Volume 2, Pages 317–323, March 12, 2018.
https://www.nature.com/articles/s41550-018-0413-4

116. How did Earth get its water?, The answer lies in deuterium ratios and a theory called the Grand Tack by Christopher Crockett, Posted on May 6, 2015.
https://www.sciencenews.org/article/how-did-Earth-get-its-water

117. Earth's Water Explained by Gas Giant Gluttony by James Romero, Posted on Jul 19, 2017.
http://www.sci-news.com/space/Earths-water-gas-giant-gluttony-05054.html

118. Journal Publication
Origin of water in the inner Solar System: Planetesimals scattered inward during Jupiter and Saturn's rapid gas accretion. Authors: Sean N. Raymond, Andre Izidoro.
Icarus, 297, 134-148 (2017), DOI: 10.1016/j.icarus.2017.06.030
https://arxiv.org/abs/1707.01234

119. List of Publications & CV of Sean Raymond
http://perso.astrophy.u-bordeaux.fr/SRaymond/

WATER FORMATION OCCURRED IN INTERSTELLAR MEDIUM
EARTH GOT ITS WATER EVEN BEFORE OUR SOLAR SYSTEM WAS BORN

120. Interstellar Medium, from Wikipedia.
https://en.wikipedia.org/wiki/Interstellar_medium

121. Five amazing facts about interstellar space by Jonathan O'Callaghan, Posted on September 13, 2013.
https://www.spaceanswers.com/deep-space/five-amazing-facts-about-interstellar-space/

122. What is interstellar space? Where does interstellar space begin?
https://spaceplace.nasa.gov/interstellar/en/

123. Interstellar Medium, Science Daily.
https://www.sciencedaily.com/terms/interstellar_medium.htm

124. The Interstellar Medium, An Online Tutorial, University of New Hampshire.
http://www-ssg.sr.unh.edu/ism/what.html
http://www-ssg.sr.unh.edu/ism/when.html
http://www-ssg.sr.unh.edu/ism/where.html
http://www-ssg.sr.unh.edu/ism/why.html
http://www-ssg.sr.unh.edu/ism/how.html

125. What is Interstellar Medium? From the Website of NASA.
https://www.nasa.gov/mission_pages/ibex/IBEXDidYouKnow.html

126. Interstellar Medium (ISM), Chapter 18
http://www.as.utexas.edu/astronomy/education/fall09/scalo/secure/301F09.Ch18.ISM.Notes.pdf

127. Interstellar Medium and the Milky Way Galaxy by Nick Strobel, Physical Science Dept., Bakersfield College, Bakersfield, CA, USA.
http://www.jb.man.ac.uk/distance/exploring/course/strobel/ismnotes/ismglxya.htm

WATER FOUND IN THE INTERSTELLAR MEDIUM (ISM)

128. Book Title: Giant Planets of Our Solar System: An Introduction by Patrick G. J. Irwin, Pages 18-19. Website Link

129. A Could of Water in Interstellar Space by Cornell University, Ithaca, NY, USA.
https://www.eurekalert.org/pub_releases/1998-04/CUNS-ACOW-090498.php

130. INFO 12-1998: ISO finds a very steamy cloud in interstellar space, Posted on April 10, 1998, Updated on May 25, 2005.
http://sci.esa.int/iso/12729-info-12-1998-iso-finds-a-very-steamy-cloud-in-interstellar-space/

131. Cold Clouds and Water in Space by Astrobiology Magazine, Posted on Jun 4, 2001.
https://www.astrobio.net/cosmic-evolution/cold-clouds-and-water-in-space/

132. Dusty experiments are solving interstellar water mystery
http://www.ras.org.uk/search/article-archive/1785-dusty-experiments-are-solving-interstellar-water-mystery

133. PhD Thesis of Victiria Frankland, School of Engineering & Physical Sciences, Heriot-Watt University, Edinburgh, Scotland.
http://www.ros.hw.ac.uk/bitstream/handle/10399/2468/FranklandV_0911_eps.pdf?sequence=1&isAllowed=y

INTERSTELLAR MEDIUM IS WHERE WATER FORMATION OCCURRED

134. Water in Interstellar Space by Nancy Atkinson, Article Written on May 6, 2008, Updated on Dec 24, 2015.
https://www.Universetoday.com/14075/water-in-interstellar-space/

135. Journal Publication (Publication Date: April 2012)
Water Formation through a Quantum Tunneling Surface Reaction, OH + H$_2$, at 10 K.
Authors: Oba, Y.; Watanabe, N.; Hama, T.; Kuwahata, K.; Hidaka, H.; Kouchi, A.
The Astrophysical Journal, Volume 749, Issue 1, article id. 67, 12 pp. (2012).
http://adsabs.harvard.edu/abs/2012ApJ...749...67O

136. Journal Publication
Experimental evidence for water formation on interstellar dust grains by hydrogen and oxygen atoms.
Authors: F. Dulieu, L. Amiaud, E. Congiu, J-H. Fillion, E. Matar, A. Momeni, V. Pironello, J. L. Lemaire, Journal of Astronmy & Astrophysics, Volume 512, March-April 2010.
https://www.aanda.org/articles/aa/full_html/2010/04/aa12079-09/aa12079-09.html

137. Complete Paper, PDF File.
https://www.aanda.org/articles/aa/pdf/2010/04/aa12079-09.pdf

138. ON WATER FORMATION IN THE INTERSTELLAR MEDIUM: LABORATORY STUDY OF THE O+D REACTION ON SURFACES, Authors: Dapeng Jing, Jiao He, John Brucato, Antonio De Sio, Lorenzo Tozzetti, and Gianfranco Vidali, The American Astronomical Society.
The Astrophysical Journal Letters, Volume 741, Number 1, October 10 2011.
http://iopscience.iop.org/article/10.1088/2041-8205/741/1/L9

EARTH INHERITED ITS WATER FROM INTERSTELLAR MEDIUM

139. Much of Earth's Water Is Older Than the Sun by Mike Wall, Senior Writer, Posted on September 25, 2014.
https://www.space.com/27256-Earth-water-older-than-sun.html

140. Half of Earth's Water Formed Before Sun Was Born by Daniel Clery, Sept 25, 2014.
http://www.sciencemag.org/news/2014/09/half-Earths-water-formed-sun-was-born

141. The water in your bottle might be older than the sun by EarthSky in Earth, Posted on September 27, 2014.
http://Earthsky.org/space/the-water-in-your-bottle-might-be-older-than-the-sun

142. The Water On Earth Predates The Formation Of The Sun by IFL Science.
http://www.iflscience.com/space/solar-systems-water-predates-sun/

143. About Half of the Water You Drink is Older than the Sun by Rick Pantaleo, Science World, Posted on September 26, 2014.
https://blogs.voanews.com/science-world/2014/09/26/about-half-of-the-water-you-drink-is-older-than-the-sun/

144. Earth's water older than the sun, came from interstellar ice by Michelle Starr, Posted on September 25, 2014.
https://www.cnet.com/news/Earths-water-older-than-the-sun-came-from-interstellar-ice/#

145. Origin of water in the solar system is interstellar by Michael Küffmeier, Astrobites, Posted on Dec 9, 2014.
https://astrobites.org/2014/12/09/origin-of-water-in-the-solar-system-is-interstellar/

146. The Water On Earth Predates The Formation Of The Sun by IFL Science.
http://www.iflscience.com/space/solar-systems-water-predates-sun/

147. Water On Earth Is Older Than Our Sun, Posted on September 25, 2014.
http://astrobiology.com/2014/09/water-on-Earth-is-older-than-our-sun.html

148. Journal Publication
Publication Title: The ancient heritage of water ice in the solar system. Authors: L. Ilsedore Cleeves, Edwin (Ted) A. Bergin, Conel M. O'D. Alexander, Fujun Du, Dawn Graninger, Karin I. Öberg, Tim J. Harries, University of Michigan, Carnegie DTM Harvard-Smithsonian CfA, University of Exeter, Science, Vol. 345 no. 6204 pp. 1590-1593, Submitted on 25 Sep 2014, Published in 2014.
https://arxiv.org/abs/1409.7398

EARTH GOT ITS WATER EVEN BEFORE THE MOON FORMATION

149. Earth had water even before the collision that made the moon, by New Scientist Staff and Press Association, Daily News, March 28, 2018.
https://www.newscientist.com/article/2165141-Earth-had-water-even-before-the-collision-that-made-the-moon/

150. How Was Water First Formed On Earth?, Quora, Discussion Forum.
https://www.quora.com/How-was-water-first-formed-on-Earth

PRIMORDIAL WATER FOUND IN EARTH'S DEEP MANTLE

151. University of Hawaii Researchers Shed New Light on the Origins of Earth's Water.
http://www.ifa.hawaii.edu/info/press-releases/water-origins/

152. How Was Water First Formed On Earth?, Quora, Discussion Forum by Anik Patni.
https://www.quora.com/How-was-water-first-formed-on-Earth

153. New Light Shed on the Origins of Earth's Water by Na Kilo Hoku, The One Who Look At The Stars.
https://www2.ifa.hawaii.edu/newsletters/article.cfm?a=766&n=61

154. Earth's Water May Be as Old as the Earth Itself, by Sarah Zielinski, Posted on November 12, 2015.
https://www.smithsonianmag.com/science-nature/Earths-water-may-be-old-Earth-itself-180957262/

155. A New Study Challenges Assumptions About the Origins of Earth's Water by Maddie Stone, Posted on Nov 14, 2015.
https://gizmodo.com/a-new-study-challenges-assumptions-about-the-origins-of-1742474825

156. Researchers shed new light on the origins of Earth's water, University of Hawaii at Manoa, Posted on November 12, 2015.
https://phys.org/news/2015-11-Earth.html

157. Earth's Oceans Have Always Been Local by Brian Koberlein, Posted on November 23, 2015.
https://briankoberlein.com/2015/11/23/local-ocean/

158. Where Did Earth's Water Come From? by Jesse Emspak, Live Science Contributor, Posted on July 7, 2016.
https://www.livescience.com/33391-where-did-water-come-from.html

159. Journal Publication
Evidence for primordial water in Earth's deep mantle. Authors: Lydia J. Hallis, Gary R. Huss, Kazuhide Nagashima, G. Jeffrey Taylor, Sæmundur A. Halldórsson, David R. Hilton, Michael J. Mottl., Science, Vol. 350, Issue 6262, pp. 795-797, 13 Nov 2015.
http://science.sciencemag.org/content/350/6262/795
https://www.researchgate.net/publication/283752386_Evidence_for_primordial_water_in_Earth%27s_deep_mantle

EARTH'S DEEP MANTLE IS RESPONSIBLE

160. There's as much water in Earth's mantle as in all the oceans by Andy Coghlan, Daily News, Posted on June 12, 2017.
https://www.newscientist.com/article/2133963-theres-as-much-water-in-Earths-mantle-as-in-all-the-oceans/

161. Journal Publication: A nearly water-saturated mantle transition zone inferred from mineral viscosity. Authors: Hongzhan Fei, Daisuke Yamazaki, Moe Sakurai, Nobuyoshi Miyajima, Hiroaki Ohfuji, Tomoo Katsura and Takafumi Yamamoto, Science Advances, Vol. 3, no. 6, e1603024, DOI: 10.1126/sciadv.1603024, 07 Jun 2017.
http://advances.sciencemag.org/content/3/6/e1603024

THICK HYDROGEN LAYER IS RESPONSIBLE

162. Earth's water brewed at home, not in space by Hazel Muir, Daily News, Posted on September 25, 2007.
https://www.newscientist.com/article/dn12693-Earths-water-brewed-at-home-not-in-space/

163. Journal Publication, Origin of the Ocean on the Earth: Early Evolution of Water D/H in a Hydrogen-rich Atmosphere. Authors: Hidenori Genda, Masahiro Ikoma, Paper Submitted on Sep 13, 2007. Journal Reference: Icarus 194:42-52,2008. https://arxiv.org/abs/0709.2025

YOUTUBE VIDEOS REGADING WATER FORMATION

164. YouTube Title: Where did Earth's water come from? Narrated by Zachary Metz, TED-Ed Lessons, Published on Mar 23, 2015.
https://www.youtube.com/watch?v=RwtO04EXgUE
165. YouTube Title: Where Did Earth's Water Come From? by MinuteEarth, Published on Feb 7, 2014.
https://www.youtube.com/watch?v=_LpgBvEPozk
166. YouTube Title: How Did Earth Get Its Water? by SciShow Space, Published on May 31, 2016.
https://www.youtube.com/watch?v=_Y-XUAKTAkE

The references from 167 to 177 are not assigned and not being used.

FORMATION OF LIFE ON OUR PLANET EARTH

178. YouTube Title: Whole Story from the Big Bang to the Present Day - Full Documentary (History of the World in 2 Hours) by Perfect Toys, Published on Apr 24, 2016. Narrators: Alex Filippenko (Astrophysicist), Peter Ward (Paleontologist), Clifford V. Johnson (Physicist, University of Southern California), and others.
https://www.youtube.com/watch?v=_ITHx8SKD5g (This video is unavailable now!)
179. History of the World in 2 Hours by Alex Filippenko (Astrophysicist), Peter Ward (Paleontologist), and others, DVD, ASIN: B006ENHGLS, Available on Amazon.com.

EVOLUTION OF LIFE AND THE ORIGIN OF LIFE

180. Human Evolution Based On Recorded Facts, Science Clarified.
http://www.scienceclarified.com/He-In/Human-Evolution.html
181. Lucy (Australopithecus), From Wikipedia, the Free Encyclopedia,
Lucy Skeleton Reconstruction at the Cleveland Museum of Natural History.
https://en.wikipedia.org/wiki/Lucy_(Australopithecus)
182. Seven (7) Theories on the Origin of Life by Charles Q. Choi, Live Science Contributor, Posted on March 24, 2016. https://www.livescience.com/13363-7-theories-origin-life.html

ARE WE ALL REALLY MADE OF STARDUST?

183. Extraordinary and Inspiring Facts About the Universe by Alex Morris.
https://www.lifehack.org/articles/lifestyle/20-extraordinary-and-inspiring-facts-about-the-Universe.html
184. Where Your Elements Came From? By Nasa.gov. Last updated March 28, 2019.
https://science.nasa.gov/where-your-elements-came
185. Dr. Carl Sagan, "Cosmos," Paperback, Ann Druyan (Introduction), Neil deGrasse Tyson (Foreword), ISBN number 9780345539434, Amazon.com, December 10, 2013.
186. Amazing Facts About our Universe You Won't Believe by Carl Pettit, Posted on November 14, 2012.   https://thefw.com/facts-about-the-universe/
187. Understanding the Evolution of Life in the Universe, Webmaster: Britt Griswold, NASA Official: Dr. Edward J. Wollack, Page Updated on Feb 26,2016.
https://wmap.gsfc.nasa.gov/universe/uni_life.html

188. Composition of the human body, From Wikipedia, the free encyclopedia.
https://en.wikipedia.org/wiki/Composition_of_the_human_body#:~:text=Almost%2099%25%20of%20the%20mass,11%20are%20necessary%20for%20life.
189. The Chemistry of Life: The Human Body by Michael Schirber, Posted on April 16, 2009.
https://www.livescience.com/3505-chemistry-life-human-body.html

<table>
<tr><td colspan="3">In CHAPTER 1 & CHAPTER 20,
You Have Learned All About
The Origin of the Earth's Water</td></tr>
</table>

● The Big Bang Theory explained in Chapter 1 of the book "Drinking Water Guide" is the most relevant, most essential, and most important part. This book teaches that all those heavier elements of our periodic table, including all those minerals that we use today to remineralize and alkalize the purified water, were originally manufactured in the burning cores of collapsing stars by a process known as "stellar nucleosynthesis," even before our Solar System and our planet Earth were created. Stars are responsible for all the constituents of our planet Earth (Carbon, Hydrogen, Nitrogen, Oxygen, Phosphorus and Sulfur are the most important elements) that are needed for the formation and survival of every human being, animal and plant.
In the Remaining Part of This Book, You Will Learn Water Statistics, Types of Drinking Water, Importance of Drinking Water, and How to Drink Only Purified Water That is Properly Remineralized and Slightly Alkalized.
Purified water (zero water) that is either neutralized (pH=7) or slightly alkalized (pH= 7 to 7.5), and remineralized up to a TDS level of 200 ppm is the healthy drinking water.

CHAPTER 2 DRINKING WATER FACTS & STATISTICS

TABLE OF CONTENTS

Facts and Statistics Posted by Water For People [1]

- 2.1 billion people around the world don't have access to safe water.
- 4.5 billion lack access to adequate sanitation.
- Women and children spend more than 4 hours walking for water each day.
- More than 840,000 people die each year from water-related diseases.

The aforementioned numbers are based off the following data:
- UNC Water Institute Study
- World Health Organization (WHO)
- National Center for Biotechnology Information (NCBI)

Facts and Statistics Posted by Water Aid [2]

- About 844 million people don't have clean water (WHO Report 2017).
  WHO = World Health Organization.

- About 2.3 billion people don't have a decent toilet (WHO Report 2017).

- About 31% of schools don't have clean water (UNICEF Report 2015).
  UNICEF = United Nations Children's Fund
         (formerly, United Nations International Children's Emergency Fund).

- About 443 million school days are lost every year because of water-related illnesses.

- Every minute a newborn dies from infection caused by lack of safe water and an unclean environment. (WHO Report 2015).

- Diarrhea (also spelled diarrhoea), caused by dirty water and poor toilets kills a child under 5 every 2 minutes. (WASHWatch.org Report).

- Every $1 invested in water and toilets returns an average of $4 in increased productivity.

- The World Bank says promoting good hygiene is one of the most cost effective health interventions.

- If everyone, everywhere had clean water, the one-third of the number of diarrhoeal (relating to diarrhea) deaths would be prevented.

Drinking Water Statistics Posted by WHO in 2018 [3]

◉ About 844 million people lack even a basic drinking-water service, including 159 million people who are dependent on surface water.

◉ Globally, at least 2 billion people use a drinking water contaminated with faeces. Contaminated water can transmit water-borne diseases such as "diarrhea (also spelled diarrhoea), cholera, polio, typhoid, and dysentery". Contaminated drinking water is estimated to cause 502,000 diarrhea deaths each year.

◉ By 2025, half of the world's population will be living in water-stressed areas. In low and middle income countries, 38% of health care facilities lack an improved water source, 19% do not have improved sanitation, and 35% lack water and soap for handwashing.

◉ In 2015, 5.2 billion people used safely managed drinking-water services. The remaining 2.1 billion people without safely managed services in 2015 included:

   ⟫ 1.3 billion people with basic services, meaning an improved water source located within a round trip of 30 minutes.

   ⟫ 263 million people with limited services, or an improved water source requiring more than 30 minutes to collect water.

   ⟫ 423 million people taking water from unprotected wells and springs.

   ⟫ 159 million people collecting untreated surface water from lakes, ponds, rivers and streams. Sharp geographic, sociocultural and economic inequalities persist, not only between rural and urban areas but also in towns and cities where people living in low-income, informal, or illegal settlements usually have less access to improved sources of drinking-water than other residents.

◉ In 2013 to 2014, water-borne diseases caused 289 cases of illnesses, 108 hospitalizations, and 17 deaths in the United States alone. As many as 63 million people from rural central California to the boroughs of New York City were exposed to potentially unsafe water more than once during the past decade. Industrial dumping, farming pollution, and pipe deterioration are the main causes of the contaminated water. In some instances it took nearly two years for the issues causing the contaminated water to be resolved.

Drinking Water Statistics Posted by New York Times [4, 5]

◉ 35 years after the U.S. Congress passed the Safe Drinking Water Act, some regulators and environmentalists state the law is now so obsolete that it fails to protect people from the most obvious threats.

◉ In the USA, the NY Times reported on violations of the Clean Water Act, a federal law which governs water pollution, and has shown household water that is contaminated with lead, nickel, and other heavy metals. Some extreme side-effects of this contamination have resulted in skin burns, rashes, and eroded tooth enamel.

⊕ The Times interviewed more than 250 state and federal regulators, water-system managers, environmental advocates and scientists. That research showed that an estimated 1 in 10 Americans have been exposed to drinking water that contains dangerous chemicals or fails to meet a federal health benchmark in other ways.

⊕ An estimated 19.5 million Americans fall ill each year from drinking water contaminated with parasites, bacteria or viruses, according to a study published last year in the scientific journal Reviews of Environmental Contamination and Toxicology. That figure does not include illnesses caused by other chemicals and toxins.

⊕ The NY Times has compiled a database of violations of the Safe Drinking Water Act, finding 40% of the nation's community water systems in violation at least once, exposing millions to potentially harmful chemicals, toxins, and heavy metals. More than 23 million people received drinking water from municipal systems that violated a health-based standard. State officials noted that they had cited more than 4,200 water pollution violations at mine sites around the state since 2000.

⊕ Chemical factories, manufacturing plants and other workplaces have violated water pollution laws more than half a million times in the past 5 years. The violations range from failing to report emissions to dumping toxins at concentrations regulators say might contribute to cancer, birth defects and other illnesses.

⊕ In the nation's largest dairy states, like Wisconsin and California, farmers have sprayed liquefied animal feces onto fields, where it has seeped into wells, causing severe infections. Tap water in parts of the Farm Belt, including cities in Illinois, Kansas, Missouri and Indiana, has contained pesticides at concentrations that some scientists have linked to birth defects and fertility problems.

⊕ In parts of New York, Rhode Island, Ohio, California and other states where sewer systems cannot accommodate heavy rains, untreated human waste has flowed into rivers and washed onto beaches. Drinking water in parts of New Jersey, New York, Arizona and Massachusetts shows some of the highest concentrations of tetrachloroethylene, a dry cleaning solvent that has been linked to kidney damage and cancer.

⊕ Records analyzed by The Times indicate that the Clean Water Act has been violated more than 506,000 times since 2004, by more than 23,000 companies and other facilities, according to reports submitted by polluters themselves. Companies sometimes test what they are dumping only once a quarter, so the actual number of days when they broke the law is often far higher. And some companies illegally avoid reporting their emissions.

⊕ In 46 states of USA, local regulators have primary responsibility for crucial aspects of the Clean Water Act. Though the number of regulated facilities has more than doubled in the last 10 years, many state enforcement budgets have remained essentially flat when adjusted for inflation. In New York, for example, the number of regulated polluters has almost doubled to 19,000 in the last decade, but the number of inspections each year has remained about the same.

⊕ Three coal companies — Loadout, Remington Coal and Pine Ridge, a subsidiary of Peabody Energy, one of the largest coal companies in the world — reported to state officials that 93% of the waste they injected near this community had illegal concentrations of chemicals including arsenic, lead, chromium, beryllium or nickel.

• More than 350 other companies and facilities in West Virginia have also violated the Clean Water Act in recent years, records show. Those infractions include releasing illegal concentrations of iron, manganese, aluminum and other chemicals into lakes and rivers.

• Department officials say they continue to improve the agency's procedures, and note that regulators have assessed $14.7 million in state fines against more than 70 mining companies since 2006.

Water-Borne Diseases [6, 7]

Water-borne diseases are developed due to contaminated water and lack of sanitation. Water-borne diseases are the leading cause of death around the world, and it's almost inexcusable on the part of local governments and municipalities. The following are the most common water-borne diseases being faced around the world:

a. Diarrhea (also spelled diarrhoea): Diarrhea is a symptom of infection caused by a host of bacterial, viral and parasitic organisms most of which can be spread by contaminated water. It is more common when there is a shortage of clean water for drinking, cooking and cleaning and basic hygiene is important in prevention. Water contaminated with human faeces for example from municipal sewage, septic tanks and latrines is of special concern. Animal faeces also contain microorganisms that can cause diarrhoea. Diarrhoea can also spread from person to person, aggravated by poor personal hygiene. Food is another major cause of diarrhoea when it is prepared or stored in unhygienic conditions. Water can contaminate food during irrigation, and fish and seafood from polluted water may also contribute to the disease.

b. Malaria: When you think of malaria you probably think of mosquitos, but malaria is also a water-borne disease. Malaria is a life threatening illness that causes high fever, chills, vomiting, and even the state of coma.

c. Cholera: Cholera is an infection of the small intestine or bowels that, if left untreated, can be fatal. Cholera typically can be contracted from infected water supplies and causing severe vomiting, diarrhea and often death. Diarrhea may seem harmless enough, but believe it or not, in developing countries without access to modern medicine and clean drinking water, cholera kills about 2.2 million people per year, usually due to severe dehydration.

d. Polio (short for Poliomyelitis): Polio is a serious infectious water-borne disease that can cause permanent paralysis (being unable to move the or body body parts).

e. Typhoid: Typhoid is an infectious bacterial fever with an eruption of red spots on the chest and abdomen and severe intestinal irritation. Contaminated water is blamed to cause this disease.

e. Dysentery: Dysentery is an infection of the intestines resulting in severe diarrhea with the presence of blood and mucus in the feces.

Keeping our water safe and clean to prevent the spread of disease should be a high priority. It's very important to clean the water that has been contaminated and keep the safe environment. Point-of-use water and sanitation technologies reduce the number of deaths caused by water-borne diseases.

Water and Sanitation [8, 9, 10]

Water sanitation is the key factor in preventing the water-borne diseases and keeping the adequate conditions for safe water supply. Water sanitation measures at any given public water supply facility include the development, application and maintenance of sanitary measures for the sake of cleanliness, protecting health, etc. Major attention should be given to maintaining clean toilets, urinary devices, sinks, showers in bathrooms, maintaining clean swimming pools, piped water to the house or yard, public taps or standpipes, boreholes, protected dug wells, protected springs and rainwater collection tanks, etc. It is very important to take responsibility is installing the systems for taking and recycling the dirty water and other waste products away from buildings in order to protect people's health. Lack of sanitation is the world's biggest cause of infection. Hand washing reduces the risk of disease by 50%. (The Global Public-Private, globalhandwashing.org, Health Impact).

The water and sanitation crisis claims more lives through disease than any war claims through guns. (United Nations Development Programme (UNDP), Human Development Report 2006, Beyond Scarcity: Power, Poverty, and the Global Water Crisis, UNDP, 2006).

At any given time, half of the world's hospital beds are occupied by patients suffering from a water-related disease. (UNICEF/WHO, Progress on Drinking Water and Sanitation: Special Focus on Sanitation, UNICEF/WHO, 2008).

Contaminants Found in Drinking Water [11, 12]

Drinking water supplies in the United States are among the safest in the world. However, according to Centers for Disease Control and Prevention (CDC), even in the USA, drinking water sources can become contaminated. In particular, people on well water in rural areas could have a higher risk of health impacts from contaminants in their tap water, making regular testing important. In developing countries, water contamination is a more serious problem.

Contaminants can be classifies into several categories:
a. Organics,
b. Inorganics,
c. Heavy Metals,
d. Fecal Matter (Cysts), and
e. Legionella.

Organics: The word organic refers to carbon-based chemicals including solvents, pesticides, and insecticides that make their way into our water through cropland runoff and factory discharge.

Inorganics: Inorganics are compounds lacking a carbon atom in their molecular structure. There are very many chemical contaminants in drinking water called inorganics. Examples include chlorine, boron, and cyanide.

Heavy Metals: Lead, Aluminum, Arsenic are the leading contaminants in drinking water. The lead particles leached out of old pipes in cities like Flint, MI and Sacramento, CA, and caused serious contamination problems.

Fecal Matter/Cysts: Microbial cysts from both human and animal fecal matter, the resting or dormant state of microorganisms, can be lurking in your drinking water. Examples would be cryptosporidium and/or giardia lambia (generally found in rural wells). They also cause gastrointestinal illnesses and cramps from long-term exposure. In 1993 there was a huge outbreak of cryptosporidium in Milwaukee Wisconsin in which 1.6 million residents became ill, and 104 people died as a result.

Legionella: The legionella bacteria are actually a naturally occurring contaminant in water, which can lead to Legionnaires' disease (a type of serious lung infection). While it's normally spread through tiny water droplets in the air, usually in buildings with larger plumbing systems, it can make it's way into your body by aspiration of drinking water if the water passes through wrong pipelines. The legionella bacteria very often affects seniors, smokers, or those with a chronic lung condition or weakened immune system.

REFERENCES

1. Safe Water and Sanitation for Generations by Water for People.
https://www.waterforpeople.org/

2. Facts and Statistics by Water Aid.
https://www.wateraid.org/facts-and-statistics

3. Drinking Water Statistics by World Health Organization (WHO), Posted on Feb 07, 2018.
http://www.who.int/news-room/fact-sheets/detail/drinking-water
http://www.who.int/en/news-room/fact-sheets/detail/drinking-water

4. Clean Water Laws Are Neglected, at a Cost in Suffering by Charles Duhiggsept by Charles Duhigg, New York Times, Posted on Sept 12, 2009.
http://www.nytimes.com/2009/09/13/us/13water.html?_r=2&pagewanted=all

5. Find Water Polluters Near You, Toxic Water, New York Times by Charles Duhigg, Posted on May 16, 2012.
http://projects.nytimes.com/toxic-waters/polluters
https://www.nytimes.com/interactive/projects/toxic-waters/polluters/index.html
https://www.nytimes.com/2009/09/13/us/13water.html

6. Water Sanitation Hygiene, Water-related Diseases, WHO Report.
http://www.who.int/water_sanitation_health/diseases-risks/diseases/diarrhoea/en/

7. Critical Facts About Water-borne Diseases In The United States and Abroad, by John Hawthorne, Posted on Feb 15, 2018.
https://businessconnectworld.com/2018/02/15/critical-facts-water-borne-diseases-us/

8. Global Water Poverty Facts by Watering Malawi.
http://wateringmalawi.org/global-water-poverty-facts/

9. Water, Sanitation and Hygiene, Global Health Observatory Data (GHO).
http://www.who.int/gho/phe/water_sanitation/en/

10. Water, Sanitation and Hygiene by UNICEF.
https://www.unicef.org/wash/

11. How to Distill Water by Pure Water, Posted on May 04, 2017
https://mypurewater.com/blog/2017/05/04/how-to-distill-water/

12. Common Contaminants Found in Drinking Water by Jeff Hayward, Posted on November 14, 2016.
https://www.activebeat.co/your-health/7-common-contaminants-found-in-drinking-water/?streamview=all

CHAPTER 3 IMPORTANCE OF DRINKING WATER

TABLE OF CONTENTS

AMAZING FACTS ABOUT WATER AND DRINKING WATER

Water On Our Planet Earth [1, 2, 3]

⚫Our beautiful and wonderful planet Earth is the third rotating and revolving planet from the Sun, and is the only astronomical object known to harbor life in our Solar System. Based on the radiometric dating and other sources of evidence, astronomers and scientists confirmed that our planet Earth is 4.54 billion years old. [1] Our planet Earth has a surface area of approximately 510 million square kilometers or 196.9 million square miles. [2]

⚫Water on our planet Earth is very abundant. About 71 percent of Earth's surface is covered by water. According to NASA's report, there are more than 326 million trillion gallons of water on Earth. [3]

⚫The oceans of our planet Earth contain about 96.5 percent of all the planet's water. Less than 3 percent of all water on Earth is freshwater (usable for drinking). More than two-thirds of Earth's freshwater is locked up in ice caps and glaciers. [3]

Human Body Is Made Up Of Water and Needs Water [4, 5, 6, 7, 8]

⚫Water is the primary molecule required and the most important ingredient necessary for the formation of life on the planet Earth. The average human adult male is approximately 60% water (by weight) and the average adult female is approximately 55% (by weight). [4]

⚫99% of Your Body's Molecules Are Water Molecules: [5a, 5b]

Scientists have determined that a typical teenager's body with 57 Kg (127 Pounds) of body weight has the following composition: 61 % water, 16 % fat, 16 % protein, 6% minerals, and 1% carbohydrate. Scientists also estimated that the same body consists of 1.2×10^{25} molecules, and more than 99% of them are water molecules. [5a, 5b]

⚫Every part of your body from your skin to your brain relies on ample hydration to function. Up to 60% of the adult human body weight is made up of water. Women have less water in their bodies compared to men. Infants bodies have 78% to 93% water, and by the age one, the water content drops to 65%. Some organisms and plants contain up to 90% of water. Up to 85% of the brain is submerged in the water that helps feed and cushion it. A scientist H.H. Mitchell reported in the Journal of Biological Chemistry that the brain and heart are composed of 73% water, and the lungs are about 83% water, the skin contains 64% water, muscles and kidneys are 79% water, and the bones are 31% water. Even the fat contains up to 20% of water. [6]

⚫The amazing human body is composed of roughly 206 bones, 600 muscles, 10,000 nerve fibers, 2 million optic nerve fibers, 100 billion nerve cells, 30 trillion blood cells, 62,000 miles in total length of blood vessels, capillaries and arteries, and so on. All body parts, which work together round the clock, 24 hours a day and 7 days a week, possess large sums of water and need fresh and pure water every single day to survive. Every cell, tissue and organ in your body possesses water and needs fresh and pure water every single day to function correctly. [7a, 7b]

⚫Water is beneficial and vital to the life of every human being, animal and plant. To feel fit and healthy, the human body should stay hydrated all the time. When you water your plants, you watch them grow taller and greener. Exactly like that, when you drink water, water acts on your body to grow and keeps you active and healthy. [8]

● Water transports nutrients throughout the entire body, especially to the brain. Water circulates throughout the human body by transporting, dissolving, replenishing nutrients and organic matter, and at the same time by carrying away waste material. Water also is needed to regulate the activities of fluids, tissues, cells, lymph, blood and glandular secretions. The shortage of water intake overtime could result in the deficiency in cell activity and thereby chronic dehydration. [8]

● Water is essentially required in your stomach, small intestine and colon for the digestion, transportation and distribution of nutrients in and out of the body's cells, lubrication, temperature regulation, removal of wastes, etc. Water regulates body temperature precisely and aids digestion process. Large amount of water is needed to transport and digest solid foods. When you eat solid foods, you should drink a lot of water. Water is lost from your body when you urinate, sweat and even when you breath out. You should immediately replace lost water by drinking more and more water throughout the day. Just listen to your body, and whenever your body demands, you must drink water. [8]

● Every part of your body relies on ample hydration to function properly. Water lifts you up, opens your senses and makes you feel refreshed and ready to take on any activity, including even sleeping. [8]

● Water lubricates and cushions your body's bones and joints. Water helps heal quickly the joint damages. Water helps maintain muscle tone as muscles are composed primarily of water. [8]

● Water helps your kidneys and liver function properly and helps reduce the fat deposits. The kidneys need plenty of water to remove salt from the blood and to remove toxins and waste. Water lubricates all your organs so that they function at their best. Water also helps the blood from thickening. [8]

DEHYDRATION & ITS SYMPTOMS
Human Body Dehydrates and Dies Within A Few Days Without Water: [9, 10, 11, 12]

● Humans need food and water to survive. The water content by weight of the human body ranges between 42% and 75%, depending on age, health, weight and gender. The average human adult male is approximately 60% water. And 99% of your molecules are water. A human can go without food for about three weeks. Mahatma Gandhi survived 21 days of complete starvation when he went on hunger strike. But a human would typically last only three to four days without water. The maximum time an individual can go without water seems to be a week, though it depends in individual body condition.

● If we expose ourselves to a hot environment and/or vigorous exercise, the body temperature rises. The only physiological mechanism humans have to keep from overheating is sweating. Evaporation of sweat cools blood in vessels in the skin, which helps to cool the entire body. Under extreme conditions of hot environment and vigorous exercise, an adult can lose between 1 and 1.5 liters of sweat per hour. If that lost water is not replaced, the total volume of the body fluid can fall quickly and, most dangerously, blood volume may drop. If this happens, two potentially life-threatening problems arise: (i) blood pressure decreases because of the low blood volume, and (ii) sweating stops and body temperature can soar even higher. Under such conditions, death occurs quickly. Children are more susceptible to rapid overheating and dehydration because of their relatively larger skin surface-to-volume ratio. A child left in a hot car unattended or an athlete exercising hard in hot weather without drinking water can dehydrate, overheat and die in a a few hours.

Your body uses water to maintain its temperature, remove waste, and lubricate joints. Your body need water is to maintain good health. Water makes up more than half of your body weight. Your body loses water each day when you go to the bathroom, sweat, and even when you breathe out. You lose water even faster when it is really hot outside, when you walk and exercise, even if if you have fever, and even illnesses such as vomiting and diarrhea can also lead to rapid water loss. If you don't replace the water you lose throughout the day, you can become dehydrated.

The Symptoms of Dehydration Are: [12]

- Little or no urine
- Urine that is darker than usual
- Dry mouth
- Sleepiness or fatigue
- Extreme thirst, Headache, Confusion
- Dizziness or lightheaded feeling
- No tears when crying

Even the mild dehydration can negatively affect your physical performance, leading to reduced endurance. A study reported that fluid loss of 1.36% after exercise, when water is not consumed, did impair both mood and concentration, while increasing the frequency of headaches. Another study reported that mild dehydration caused by exercise or heat can negatively affect many other aspects of brain function.

How Much Water A Person Should Drink? [13, 14, 15, 16, 17]

(i) An Adult Must Drink At least 8 Cups of Water Per Day.
It is very important that you must replace water you have been losing throughout the day, by drinking a glass of water every now and then, even when you are not eating, and even when you are not thirsty. Health experts recommend that an adult must drink 8 cups or 2 liters of water per day.

1 Cup = 1 Glass = 8 Ounces = 250 mL = 1/4 Liter

According to several studies, drinking 2 cups (500 mL) of water can temporarily boost metabolism by 24-30%. Some researchers estimated that drinking 8 cups (2 liters) of water in one day can increase energy expenditure by about 96 calories per day. Drinking cold water is also recommended because your body works hard and burns calories to heat the cold water to your body temperature.

Drinking water about a half hour before meals can also reduce the amount of calories people end up consuming, especially in older individuals. One study showed that dieters who drank 500 ml of water before meals lost 44% more weight over a period of 12 weeks, compared to those who did not drink water before meals.

(ii) RESEARCH STUDY: How Much Water A Person Should Drink?
According to the research study conducted by National Academies of Sciences, Engineering and Medicine, healthy sedentary men need about 15.5 cups of fluid and women need 11.5 cups of fluid each day, and they get only about 20 percent of that fluid from daily food consumption (all natural foods contain water). [17]

(iii) Did You Know "Extreme Weight Loss Contestants" Drink 16 cups (4 Liters) of Water Per Day to Achieve Their Weight-Loss Goals?
After started drinking 16 cups of purified water (RO water) per day, the author of this book (Dr. RK) lost weight fast, and achieved his weight-loss goal.

HOW DRINKING WATER SPEEDS UP WEIGHT LOSS?

Drinking Water May Speed Up Weight Loss [18]
• Researchers in Germany found that drinking lots of water may speed up weight loss. Metabolic rate increases slightly with an increase in water consumption. After drinking approximately 17 ounces (2 cups) of water, the subjects' metabolic rates increased by 30% for both men and women.

How Does Water Flush Fat Out of Your System? [19]
• Drinking water before you eat may help you eat less. A 2010 study published on Obesity investigated the effects of drinking 2 cups of water before meals on weight loss among a group of people following a low-calorie diet. The study found that the water-drinking group lost more weight than the control group. Drinking water before you eat helps fill you up so you eat less, which may help you lose weight.

Does Water Flush Out Fat? (Discussion Forum) [20]
• Water flushes out fat cells and ketones. Hydration is extremely important for this and it also keeps our bowels working correctly. Water also flushes out water weight. It sounds stupid and does not make sense, but some of our weight is in water and by drinking water we flush out that old water weight that is sticking onto us and you actually may lose a few pounds after drinking water.

• Whether you are dieting or not, water consumption is essential for good health. You're not flushing out fat cells, but rather flushing out the waste products your body makes. Water retention becomes a serious problem and the body tends to hold onto water if there isn't enough coming into your body.

Water: How 8 Glasses A Day Keep Fat Away? [21]
• Drinking Enough Water is the Best Treatment for Fluid Retention. Water is needed in great quantities for fat metabolism and for the disposal of waste generated once fats are metabolized. When a person is obese or overweight, he/she needs more water than he/she would require with normal body weight. Water flushes away the waste. When a person loses weight (losing weight means burning fat), the body becomes very busy getting rid of a lot of waste generated due to fat metabolism.

• When water retention becomes a serious problem, you need to cut salt consumption. When you consume excess salt, your body retains more and more water to dilute the sodium. If you want to get rid of excess sodium in your system, drink plenty of water. As water is forced through the kidneys, it will remove the excess sodium.

• When you drink limited quantity of water, the body perceives that there is scarcity of water for future survival, and begins to store water in the extracellular spaces, outside the cell walls. This kind of water storage could cause swollen feet, swollen legs and swollen hands. Doctors then prescribe diuretics to their patients to force out the stored water from the extracellular spaces. But if you drink plenty of water (at least 8 glasses per day), you would not encounter such situations. Drinking plenty of water also helps constipation.

IF YOU DRINK LOTS OF WATER, YOU MUST REMINERALIZE WATER
• Drinking too much water in an attempt to lose weight could lead to dangerously low levels of sodium in your blood. Therefore when you drink more than 8 cups of purified water per day, you should learn how to remineralize and slightly alkalize the purified water at home. This book teaches "How to Remineralize and Alkalize the Purified Water at Home!" in Chapter 14, Chapter 17 & Chapter 18.

The Water Report: [22]
How 8 Glasses of Water Per Day Fights Weight Gain!

● Pure and clean water such as distilled water or RO water may be the only true Magic Potion for permanent weight loss! If you stop drinking enough water, your body fluids will again be thrown out of balance. So never stop drinking water.

DRINKING ICE-COLD WATER BURNS MORE CALORIES

● Cold water is absorbed more quickly into the system than warm water. Evidence suggests that by drinking ice-cold water a person can actually burn more calories. In order to raise the ice-cold water temperature to your normal body temperature (normal body temperature is 37°C/98.6°F), your body has to work harder and burn more calories. When your body burn more calories, you lose weight and you feel good.

● When the body gets enough water to function optimally, all the body system fluids will achieve perfect balance. As a result, the endocrine gland function improves, fluid retention is alleviated as stored water is lost, more fat can be used as fuel because the liver is free to metabolize stored fat, natural thirst to drink water returns, and there is a loss of hunger almost overnight.

DRINKING LOTS OF WATER REDUCES FAT DEPOSITS

● Kidneys cannot function properly without drinking enough water. When the kidneys do not function, the liver takes responsibility to do the kidney's job. But the liver's primary function is to metabolize stored fat into usable energy for the body. But if the liver has to do some of the kidney's work, it cannot work at full throttle. So you must drink lots of water to help your body.

DRINK ONLY PURIFIED WATER ALL THE TIME (Recommendations by Dr.RK)

● Environmental Protection Agency (EPA) began enforcing the water purification and treatment standards for municipal water systems long ago. But there continues to be incidents of contamination, which could be harmful to your health. So you cannot trust tap water even if your local municipality says that the tap water is being purified. You must take your own measures to make sure that the water you drink is indeed purified.

OPTION 1: Installing a reliable and high-quality faucet-filtration system to your kitchen sink at home is one option. And get your filtered water tested by a certified lab.
OPTION 2: Purchasing RO water or distilled water from supermarkets or local vendors is the much easier alternative option. RO water is much cheaper than distilled water.

● However, you should test the purified water every now and then and make sure that the water you drink is indeed purified, and not contaminated. You can do the following:

(i) Use a TDS meter to monitor the TDS (Total Dissolved Solids) level of purified water. The TDS level of purified water should be below 5 ppm, and the TDS level of distilled water should be precisely zero.
(ii) Use pH drops or pH meter, chlorine test kits and fluoride test kits every now and then.
(iii) Get your drinking water tested by a certified laboratory in your area at least once or twice a year.
(iv) Please also learn how to neutralize your body by consuming a lemon a day (Chapter 18).
(v) Please also learn how to neutralize or slightly alkalize, and remineralize the purified water up to a TDS level of 200 ppm. Please refer to Chapter 14, Chapter 17, Chapter 18 & Chapter 19. There are more than 10 experiments conducted at home.

● These healthy water-drinking habits would protect your health, keep you out of trouble, and save your own life and lives of all your family members.

What 8 Cups of Purified Water Per Day Would Do To Your Body?
How Drinking Water Would Help Improve Your Overall Health!

- Increases metabolism (cold water).
- Makes you feel full (warm water).
- Helps you lose weight.
- Flushes out toxins.
- Gets you healthier skin.
- Reduces risk of certain cancers.
- Helps digestion and constipation.
- Relieves fatigue and energizes.
- Improves overall health.

▷ All of the above for ZERO calories.

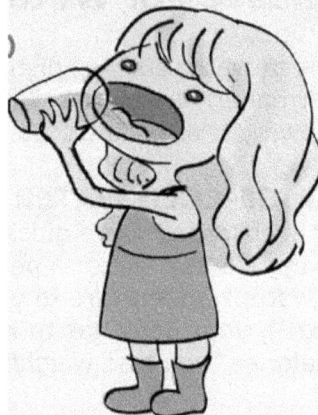

- Did you know more than 99% of your amazing body's molecules are water molecules, and 55% to 60% of your body weight is water? You therefore should make sure that the water in your body is clean, healthy and nutritious, and more importantly one 100% free of contaminants.

- So please do not drink tap water, well water, or bottled water of any kind without knowing how pure it is. Please always drink AT LEAST 8 CUPS OF PURIFIED WATER (RO water, distilled water, or zero water). And learn how to remineralize and slightly alkalize the purified water at home!

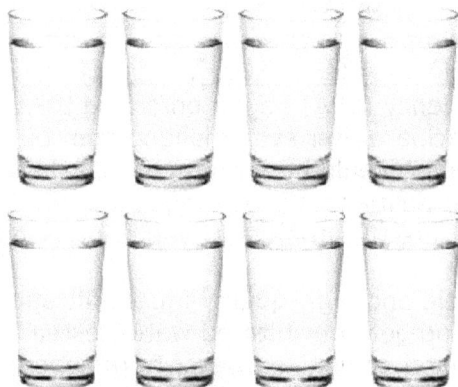

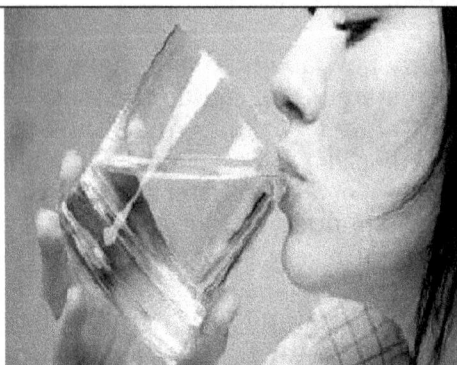

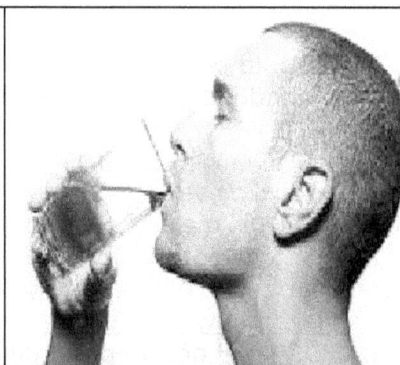

Figure 3.1 How drinking water would help improve your overall health!

REFERENCES

1. Earth, from Wikipedia, the free encyclopedia.
https://en.wikipedia.org/wiki/Earth

2. Space and Astronomy News, Universe Today, Posted on Feb 10, 2017.
https://www.universetoday.com/25756/surface-area-of-the-earth/

3. Oceans Worlds, Water in the Solar System and Beyond by NASA.
https://www.nasa.gov/specials/ocean-worlds/

4. Body water from Wikipedia, the free encyclopedia.
https://en.wikipedia.org/wiki/Body_water

5a. 99% of Your Molecules are Water by Malaga Bay, Posted on March 15, 2014.
https://malagabay.wordpress.com/2014/03/15/99-of-your-molecules-are-water/

5b. How many molecules are in the human body? by Ernest Z, Posted on June 18, 2016.
https://socratic.org/questions/how-many-molecules-are-in-the-human-body

6. The Water in You by the USGS (The United States Geological Survey) Water Science School, Contact: Howard Perlman, Posted on Dec o2, 2016.
https://water.usgs.gov/edu/propertyyou.html

7a. Permanent Diabetes Control (Book), Authored by Rao Konduru, MS, PhD, Reviewed and Endorsed by Dr. Marshal Dahl, MD, PhD., Page 31.

7b. The Amazingly Complex Human Body by Cloversites.com.
http://storage.cloversites.com/makinglifecountministriesinc/documents/Amazing%20Human%20Body_3.pdf

8. Benefits of Water, Posted by Brita.ca.
https://brita.ca/water-wellness/benefits/

9. Here's how many days a person can survive without water by Dina Spector, Posted on March 8, 2018.
http://www.businessinsider.com/how-many-days-can-you-survive-without-water-2014-5

10. How Long Can a Person Survive Without Water? by Rafi Letzter, Staff Writer, Posted on November 29, 2017.
https://www.livescience.com/32320-how-long-can-a-person-survive-without-water.html

11. How Long Can the Average Person Survive Without Water? by Randall K. Packer, a professor of biology at George Washington University, Scientific American.
https://www.scientificamerican.com/article/how-long-can-the-average/

12. Hydration: Why It Is Important by FamilyDoctor.Org.
https://familydoctor.org/hydration-why-its-so-important/

13. How much water should you drink per day? By Southwest Family Medicine Associates, Dallas, Texas, USA.
https://www.southwestfamilymed.com/blog/how-much-water-should-you-drink-per-day

14. How Much Water Does Your Body Need To Prevent Health Problems?, Posted by Gayatri Friday, May 01, 2020.
https://www.nyoooz.com/features/health/how-much-water-does-your-body-need-to-prevent-health-problems.html/3538/

15. Should You Drink 3 Liters of Water per Day? Written by Rachael Link, Healthline, Updated and Posted on June 10, 2020.
https://www.healthline.com/health/3-liters-of-water

16. Water consumption increases weight loss during a hypocaloric diet intervention in middle-aged and older adults, Randamized Study, by Elizabeth A Dennis 1, Ana Laura Dengo, Dana L Comber, Kyle D Flack, Jyoti Savla, Kevin P Davy, Brenda M Davy, Obesity (Silver Spring), 2010 Feb;18(2):300-7. doi: 10.1038/oby.2009.235. Epub 2009 Aug 6.
https://pubmed.ncbi.nlm.nih.gov/19661958/
https://www.ncbi.nlm.nih.gov/pmc/articles/PMC2859815/

17. Is alkaline water really better for you? by Christy Brissette, Posted on August 28, 2019.
https://www.washingtonpost.com/lifestyle/wellness/is-alkaline-water-really-better-for-you/2019/08/27/8c646d26-c462-11e9-b72f-b31dfaa77212_story.html

18. Drinking Water May Speed Weight Loss by WebMD.com.
http://www.webmd.com/diet/news/20040105/drinking-water-may-speed-weight-loss

19. How Does Water Flush Fat Out of Your System? by JILL CORLEONE, RDN, LD Last Updated: Jun 17, 2015.
http://www.livestrong.com/article/545311-how-does-water-flush-fat-out-of-your-system/

20. Does Water Flush Out Fat? (Discussion Forum).
http://forum.lowcarber.org/archive/index.php/t-336946.html

21. Water: How 8 Glasses A Day Keep Fat Away by Angelfire.com.
http://www.angelfire.com/ca2/LowcarbingDream/water.html

22. The Water Report: How 8 Glasses of Water per Day Fights Weight Gain! by Colon Therapists Network.
http://www.colonhealth.net/healtharticles/8-glasses-water-per-day-fights-weight-gain.html

CHAPTER 4: TYPES OF DRINKING WATER
A QUICK REVIEW

TABLE OF CONTENTS

Table 4.1 Types of drinking water available for human consumption.

TYPES OF DRINKING WATER	
Tap Water, Well Water, Even Boiled Tap Water, Bottled Water & Spring Water Are Unpurified Waters. So You Should Avoid Drinking Them.	
I. Tap Water **CHAPTER 5**	Tap water is untrustworthy although almost all local Government municipalities encourage you to drink it. You never know what contaminants are lurking in your tap water that endanger your health. Do not become another statistic! Install a high-quality faucet filter, and replace it once every 3 months or whenever the lifespan of the filter cartridge exhausts. Get your filtered water from tap tested at least once every 6 months, and make sure it is free of contaminants. Consider drinking purified water instead! As an example, read the tap water disaster story that took place recently in Flint, Michigan, USA (Chapter 5), and learn your lesson.
II. Boiled Water **CHAPTER 6**	Boiled tap water kills most of the pathogens (all kinds of bacteria, viruses, fungi, parasites), microorganisms and E. coli instantly, preventing diseases. But the harmful heavy metal and mineral contaminants such as lead, arsenic, aluminum, etc. may still remain in tap water even if it is boiled.
III. Bottled Water **(Including Vitamin Water** **and Mineral Water)** **CHAPTER 7**	Bottled water is made from tap water by adding artificial vitamins, minerals, artificial flavors, and additives. It is untrustworthy and unreliable. Testing revealed (there are many reports) that it could contain harmful chemicals, microplastics, pesticides and very many dangerous contaminants. Natural Resources Defense Council (NRDC) found that the harmful contaminants in bottled water outweigh the benefits of the filtered water. Also, bottled water is horrific for the environment and ecosystems surrounding you. Approximately only 1 in 5 plastic bottles are recycled, and those un-recycled bottles remain in the environment and it can take some 400 to 1000 years for those plastics to decompose.
IV. Spring Water **CHAPTER 8**	Spring water is bottled water. Spring water is the natural water possessing trace minerals in it, but it is not purified water. Even though it contains trace minerals, you never know what contaminants are present in it so it is untrustworthy. However, many people still like and drink spring water because of its taste and mineral composition.
V. Well Water **CHAPTER 9**	Well water is the groundwater that is reached by drilling, and then pumped to the surface. Well water in rural areas is highly contaminated. Boiled well water may minimize the risk but it still may contain dangerous heavy metal contaminants, pesticides, both human and animal feces. Get your well water tested at least once every 6 months, and filter the water with a reliable filter, and boil it before drinking.

PURIFIED WATER

Distilled Water, RO Water, Demineralized Water or Deionized Water, Desalinated Water Are Most Commonly Used Purified Waters.

Test your purified water with a TDS meter, and pH drops or digital pH meter. Make sure it is what it says on their labels. Do not be illuded by empty promises. Make sure their promises are true by testing the water. When Dr. RK tested Santevia water pitcher, it failed miserably. The pH and TDS value of filtered water were found to be unchanged from tap water. The company manager, when questioned, was found suspicious, and refused to provide any further information.

VI. Demineralized Water/Deionized Water CHAPTER 10	Both demineralization and deionization processes use "ion exchange" as the basic principle to produce purified water. This kind of water has no minerals in it. WHO warned that drinking demineralized water is harmful to your health. So you should consume well-balanced diet by eating leafy vegetables & fruits, and supplement your diet with high-quality multivitamins and minerals (magnesium, calcium, potassium, and others of your choice).
VII. Reverse Osmosis Water/RO Water CHAPTER 11 ● Purchase RO water from local vendors, or in supermarkets at Refill Yourself Stations.	It is the best "purified water" after distilled water. It is the most economical purified water available to consumers in supermarkets (a lot cheaper than buying distilled water in pharmacies). The process removes chlorine, mineral content and all other contaminants of water by forcing the water through a semi permeable membrane. This process filters out 95% to 99% of the "total dissolved solids (salts & minerals)" present in tap water. So you should consume a well-balanced diet by eating leafy vegetables & fruits, and supplement your diet with high-quality multivitamins and minerals (magnesium, calcium, potassium, and others of your choice). Please consider remineralizing the RO water with a tiny bit of Himalayan pink salt, Celtic sea salt, or ConcenTrace mineral drops in order to remineralize it (See Chapter 17).
VIII. Desalinated Water CHAPTER 12	It is the same as RO water without any minerals or trace minerals. Consider remineralizing this water, and consume balanced meals, and take supplements (vitamins and minerals).
IX. Distilled Water CHAPTER 13 ● Purchase a counter-top home distiller that makes 1 gallon of distilled water in 5.5 hours.	Distilled water is the purest form of water. This process removes one 100% of the total dissolved solids (salts and minerals). WHO reported that the distilled water lacks nutritional value (minerals) to the human health, and it could suck the minerals out of your body, if consumed for long time, causing diseases and disorders. However there is no solid scientific proof of these claims. Many people still drink the distilled water. Some people remineralize the distilled water before drinking. You will be fine if you consume a well-balanced diet and supplement with high-quality multivitamins and minerals. Please consider neutralizing your body by eating one lemon a day, and/or slightly alkalizing you body by adding a tiny pinch of baking soda to distilled water you drink.
X. ZeroWater, Brita and Pur Filtration Systems CHAPTER 14	If genuine RO water and distilled water are not available in the market, this book suggests that a consumer must switch to zero water. Make your own purified water using a ZeroWater pitcher.

	And learn how to remineralize and slightly alkalize the zero water at home. Everything is explained clearly in Chapter 14.
XI. Remineralized Water **CHAPTER 17** (A Very Important Chapter)	Purified and remineralized water, made at home, is the healthy & nutritious mineral water. Remineralized water can be obtained by adding a tiny bit of Himalayan pink salt, Celtic sea salt, or ConcenTrace mineral drops to the purified water (RO water, distilled water, or zero water) up to a TDS level of 200 ppm. Please see Chapter 17 for the experiments conducted at home, and to learn how to do it correctly. Whenever you remineralize the purified water for the first time, test it by using a TDS meter, and do not exceed the TDS level over 200 ppm. It is the best way to make and drink your own mineral water at home instead of purchasing that overpriced and dangerous "bottled mineral water ".

XII. ALKALINE WATER: CHAPTER 18
(A Very Important Chapter)

Alkaline Water Can Be Obtained by 10 Methods As Listed Below:

Purchase pH testing drops or a reliable digital pH meter to test the water pH, and learn how to neutralize, slightly alkalize and fully alkalize the purified water by adding a tiny bit of baking soda or a few ConcenTrace mineral drops.

Drinking alkaline water will help your body neutralize the acidity that it gains from different foods, juices and beverages as well as stress. Most alkaline substances become carbon dioxide and water once they are oxidized. Your body spends less energy neutralizing overly acidic substances if you drink alkaline water, and they can easily be excreted by the kidneys.

On the other hand, drinking too much alkaline water for a long term is harmful to your body as your stomach needs acidity for the digestion process and to kill bacteria. So you need to optimize the quantity of alkaline water consumption by drinking it periodically.

1. Add Lemon Juice to purified water. Lemon does not alkalize the water. The urine pH does not rise above 7 (pH < 7).	The best natural method to live healthy. Upon drinking lemon water, urine pH rises to 7 only. Lemon slightly neutralizes your body & does not alkalize. More importantly you cannot make alkaline water by adding lemon juice.
2. Add a Pinch of Baking Soda to purified water. It is perfectly alkaline water. Drinking water pH can be increased up to 8.5.	Upon adding it to purified water and drinking it, urine pH rises up to 8.5. This method has side effects (gastrointestinal distress) so make sure it suits your body.
3. Add ConcenTrace mineral drops to purified water. Drinking water can be easily alkalized.	It is very easy to remineralize and alkalize the purified water by adding only 2 drops of ConcenTrace mineral drops. Highly recommended.
4. Purchase Alkaline Water from Local vendors.	Research in your area, and find out the addresses of local vendors who sell both purified water (RO water) and alkaline water. These vendors routinely test the water and make sure that the unit is working perfectly. Therefore the water you purchase is reliable and trustworthy.

5. Purchase pH booster drops, and add to purified water. It is perfectly alkaline water. pH can be adjusted up to 9, 10, or more.	pH drops are unreliable unless the company provides the report of analysis. Drops may contain contaminants or toxins. So get your drinking water tested before you start drinking this kind of alkaline water.
6. Purchase an Alkaline Water Pitcher that adds minerals to tap water or purified water and raises water pH, making it alkaline.	Pitchers filter tap water and add minerals such as calcium, magnesium, potassium, sodium and iron. Do not believe their labels and verbal promises. Test it before using it and make sure it works by using a TDS meter and a digital pH meter. It is not reliable until you test the final product.
7. Purchase a Water Ionizer that purifies and turns your tap water to alkaline water at the touch of a button.	pH can be adjusted (8 to 11 or more). However, maintaining this kind of unit at home is tedious. You need to test drinking water every day and make sure it is working. You never know if it is working or broke down.
8. Purchase a Kangen Water Machine that turns your tap water to alkaline water and acidic water (pH adjustable).	KANGEN WATER MACHINE: Maintaining this kind of unit at home is tedious. You need to test drinking water every day and make sure it is working. You never know if the machine is working or broke down.
9. Purchase a Hydrogen Water Generator. (Not necessarily alkaline water, it could have neutral pH).	HYDROGEN WATER MACHINE: It produces either alkaline water or non-alkaline water depending on the brand name. Needs to check for H2 concentration in drinking water frequently. Again you need to test final product and make sure it is working.
10. Purchase a Reverse Osmosis System that purifies tap water, remineralizes and pours alkaline water (pH adjustable) into your jug at the touch of a button.	REVERSE OSMOSIS SYSTEM: Maintaining this kind of unit at home is tedious. You need to test drinking water every day or every now and then and make sure it is working. You never know if the machine is working or broke down. Purchase a TDS meter, and test your water for TDS level. Do not drink water with TDS > 200 ppm.

OTHER TYPES OF WATER

XIII. Water From Atmospheric Water Generators **CHAPTER 15**	Water from atmospheric air is produced through dehumidification of air. The moisture in air is cooled, captured, condensed into droplets and collected into a receiver or reservoir, which is then filtered and purified to obtain safe drinking water. You should consider remineralizing this purified water in order to comply with the WHO suggestion that drinking water should contain minimal mineral content. Also please consider neutralizing or slightly alkalizing your drinking water before consuming.

FINAL MESSAGE: Please do not drink tap water, well water, or bottled water of any kind without knowing how pure it is. Please always drink purified water that is either neutralized or slightly alkalized, and remineralized up to a TDS (Total Dissolved Solids) level of 200 ppm, which is the healthy drinking water.

Purchasing expensive water purification systems for home use is unnecessary. Learn how to purchase or make your own purified water at home. Please refer to the 2nd Part of this book (Chapter 17, Chapter 18 and Chapter 19), and learn how to remineralize and alkalize the purified water at home.

CHAPTER 14: ZEROWATER, BRITA AND PUR FILTRATION SYSTEMS TO PRODUCE PURIFIED WATER AT HOME

TABLE OF CONTENTS

ZEROWATER'S 5-STAGE ION EXCHAGE FILTRATION IN ACTION [1]

Tap water may look clean, but could pick up hidden contaminants while traveling through pipes. ZeroWater company claims that its 5-stage Ion Exchange filtration removes more dissolved solids than ANY other pour-through filter in the world. By removing 99.6% of all TDS (Total Dissolved Solids), the filter leaves nothing behind but the pure water H2O. ZeroWater filter with its advanced technology is certified to remove virtually all dissolved solids from tap water, including the most commonly found contaminants like lead, chromium, mercury, and PFOA & PFOS.

As tap water passes through five distinct sections vertically, the filter removes the visible solids, inorganic compounds, and contaminants that lurk in our tap water so that we can drink the purest tasting and contaminant-free water worry-free. The 5-stage filtration process removes everything from tap water, leaving behind zero dissolved solids as shown below:

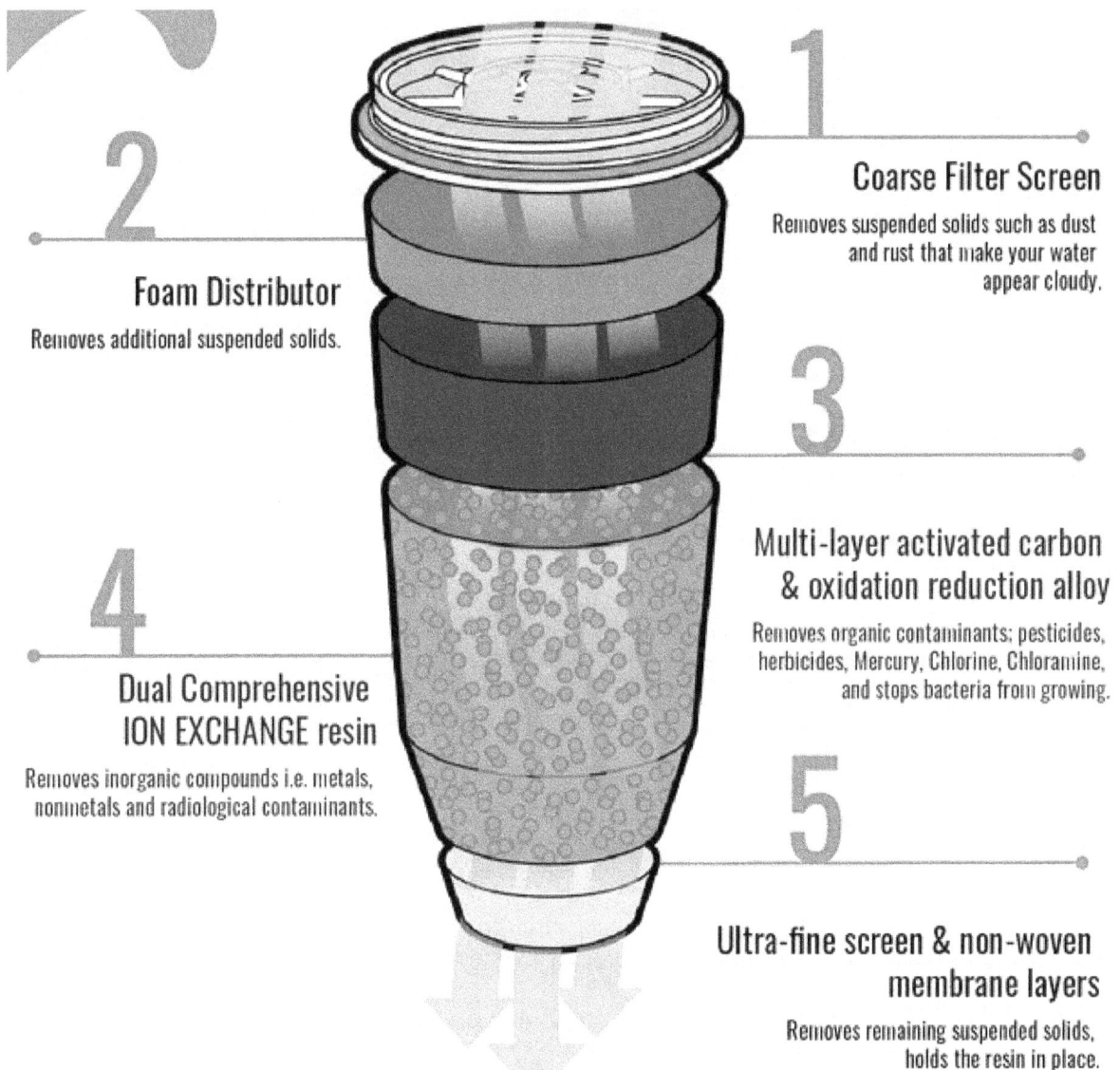

2 Foam Distributor
Removes additional suspended solids.

4 Dual Comprehensive ION EXCHANGE resin
Removes inorganic compounds i.e. metals, nonmetals and radiological contaminants.

1 Coarse Filter Screen
Removes suspended solids such as dust and rust that make your water appear cloudy.

3 Multi-layer activated carbon & oxidation reduction alloy
Removes organic contaminants; pesticides, herbicides, Mercury, Chlorine, Chloramine, and stops bacteria from growing.

5 Ultra-fine screen & non-woven membrane layers
Removes remaining suspended solids, holds the resin in place.

Courtesy of ZEROWATER
Figure 14.1 The 5-stage ZroWater filtration process is explained. [1]

WHAT ARE PFAS, PFOA & PFOS? [2]

PFAS = polyfluoroalkyl substances
PFOA = perfluorooctanoic acid
PFOS = perfluorooctane sulfonate

PFAS are a group of man-made, large, complex, and ever-expanding group of manufactured chemicals that are widely used to make various types of everyday needful products. These chemicals because of their unique ability to repel oil and water do not degrade over time, but they accumulate within the environment, and could slowly end up in the water we drink. For example, they prevent food from sticking to nonstick cookware, make clothes and carpets resistant to stains (stain repellents), and create firefighting foam that is more effective, waterproof clothing and shoes, fast food wrappers, personal care products, and many other fancy consumer goods. PFAS are vastly used in industries such as aerospace, automotive, construction, electronics, and military.

In general, there are two types of PFAS most commonly produced worldwide:
(i) PFOA (perfluorooctanoic acid) and
(ii) PFOS (perfluorooctane sulfonate)

ZeroWater filter is certified to reduce these most dangerous PFOA & PFOS, thereby making the drinking water safe.

THE SUPERIORITY OF THE ZEROWATER'S 5-STAGE FILTRATION TECHNIQUE [2, 3]

ZeroWater company (Zero Technologies, LLc) has been designing, manufacturing and marketing many 5-Stage filtration pitchers and dispensers for getting TDS free water at home or in the office. All pitchers remove 99.6% of dissolved solids, including organic and inorganic materials, such as metals, minerals, salts, and ions dissolved in water. TDS can affect the taste and appearance of water but are not harmful to consume. All pitchers and dispensers fit perfectly either on on the counter or in the refrigerator. All pitchers and dispensers come with a ZeroWater® TDS meter so that a customer can easily monitor the TDS level the zero water made using any pitcher.

ZeroWater claims that: Even if all the municipalities with superior technological advancements achieve the removal of 99.6% of total dissolved solids, the water could pick up chemicals, lead and dirt on its way from the treatment plant, through pipelines, to the faucet. Even the minute quantities of the added chlorine by municipalities is harmful to the children. The taste of the tap water may not be appreciated and the quality may not be trustworthy.

ZeroWater's products are internationally certified against NSF/ANSI standards, delivering the purest tasting water of any pour-through water filter. ZeroWater's 5-stage filtration system is far superior to the Brita filtration system in removing the following contaminants: [3]

METALS SUCH AS: ANTIMONY, ARSENIC, BARIUM, BERYLLIUM, CADMIUM, CHROMIUM, COPPER, IRON, LEAD, MANGANESE, MERCURY, SELENIUM, SILVER, THALLIUM, ZINC, and
INORGANIC NON-METALS SUCH AS: CHLORINE, CYANIDE, FLUORIDE, NITRATE, NITRITE.

The results can be seen on a comparison chart shown on the following webpage:
https://zerowater.com/pages/results

ZEROWATER PRODUCTS (PITCHERS, DISPENSERS & FAUCET FILTERS) [4]
All ZeroWater products are made from BPA-Free hard plastic so that they last longer.

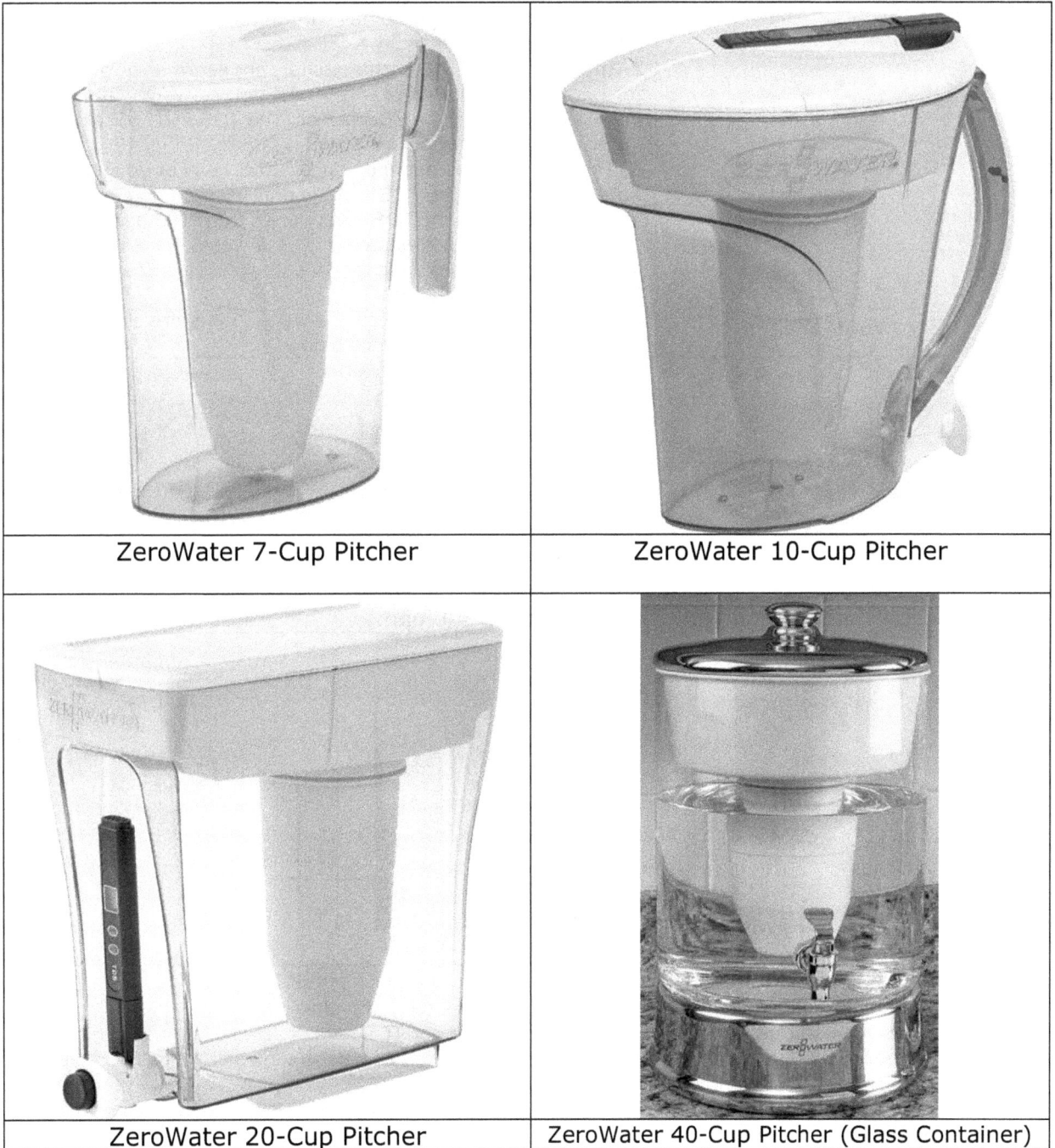

ZeroWater 7-Cup Pitcher	ZeroWater 10-Cup Pitcher
ZeroWater 20-Cup Pitcher	ZeroWater 40-Cup Pitcher (Glass Container)

FAUCET FILTERS are installed to the tip of kitchen sink faucet to remove contaminants from tap water. Faucet filters do not reduce the TDS level of tap water. The major advantage is that if you install a faucet filter to sink, the ZeroWater filter lasts longer.

Courtesy of ZEROWATER

Figure 14.2 ZeroWater 5-Stage Water Filtration Products to purify water.

HOW TO REMINERALIZE AND SLIGHTLY ALKALIZE THE ZERO WATER
(Same Procedure Can Be Used for Any Kind of Purified Water)

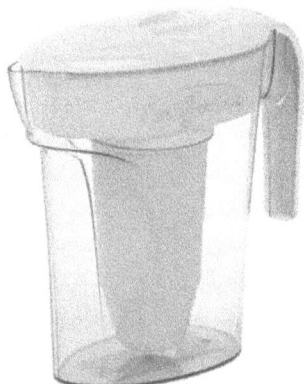

1. Purchase a ZeroWater pitcher on Zerowater.com or from any local retail store. It comes with a ZeroWater filter and also a TDS meter.

2. Install the filter inside the pitcher, and learn how to make zero water from tap water. After making zero water, monitor the TDS level using the TDS meter. The TDS level of zero water should be precisely 0 ppm.

3. The filter lifetime depends on the TDS level of your tap water. In Canada, the TDS level is only 20 ppm and so it lasts long. In USA, the TDS level varies from 100 ppm to 300 ppm so the filter is exhausted in 3 to 4 weeks for a single person if he/she drinks 8 cups of water per day. You can use the filter until TDS=5 ppm.

4. Make enough zero water for a week, and store zero water in four 4-liter bottles as show below.

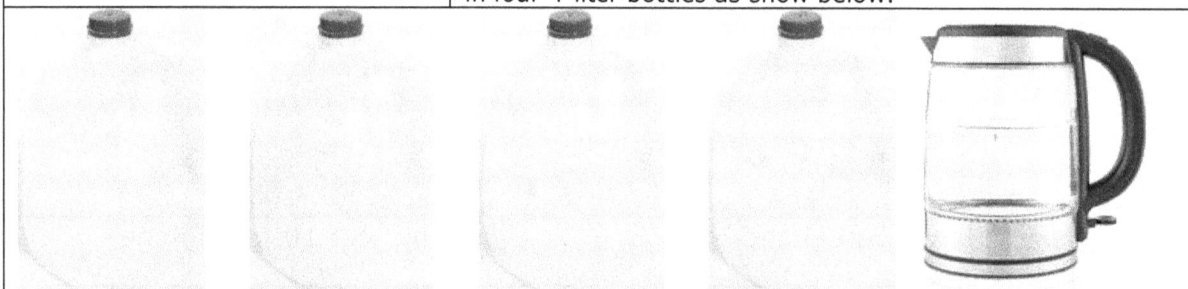

ZeroWater Pitcher

4-Liter Bottles Filled With Zero Water (TDS = 0 ppm)

Glass Kettle (1.7 Liters)

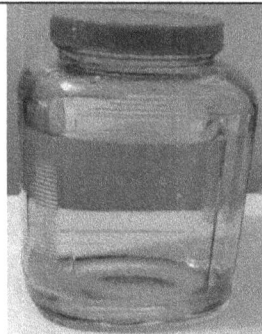

Glass Bottle Filled With 4-Liters of Zero Water

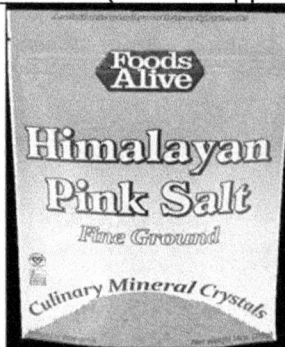

Himalayan pink salt

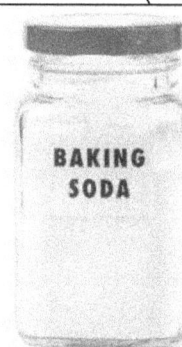

Baking Soda

5. Transfer 4 liters of zero water (you have just made) into a glass bottle.

6. Add a tiny pinch (only a few kernels) of Himalayan pink salt, and shake the bottle in a circular motion so that all water is remineralized. Monitor TDS level. Make sure that TDS is 20 ppm, 50 ppm, or 100 ppm (your desired TDS level). Add more Himalyan pink salt if the TDS level is below your desired level. Do not exceed TDS=200 ppm.

7. Add a tiny pinch of baking soda (only a few kernels), shake the bottle thoroughly and measure the pH. pH should be close to 7 (maximum 7.25).

8. Boil this remineralized and slightly alkalized zero water by using a glass kettle, store it in glass bottle until it is cooled, transfer to 4-liter plastic bottles, refrigerate it, and drink it.

9. IMPORTANT NOTE: When you use baking soda to increase the pH of the purified water, you must do urine test frequently and make sure that your urine pH is under 8.

Purified water (zero water) that is either neutralized (pH=7) or slightly alkalized (pH= 7 to 7.5), and remineralized up to a TDS level of 200 ppm is the healthy drinking water.

Figure 14.3 How to make healthy drinking water from zero water.

HOW TO USE TWO ZERO WATER FILTERS SIMULTANEOUSLY AND SAVE MONEY?

1. ZeroWater company suggests that whenever the TDS level of filtered water reaches 6 ppm, you must dispose the filter, purchase a replacement filter, and use it to produce zero water on an ongoing basis.

2. But Drinking Water Guide advises that if you use two filters simultaneously and wisely as explained here, you can save a lot of money in a long run.

3. Purchase two ZeroWater pitchers. Start using Pitcher-I until the TDS level reaches 6 ppm. Do not dispose this filter and keep using it. Store this filtered (not drinkable) water at 6 ppm to 10 ppm in 4-liter bottles as shown below.

4. Filter this water at 6 ppm in Pitcher-II, which will reduce TDS level from 6 ppm to 0 ppm. Store this filtered (drinkable) water at 0 ppm in different 4-liter bottles as shown below.

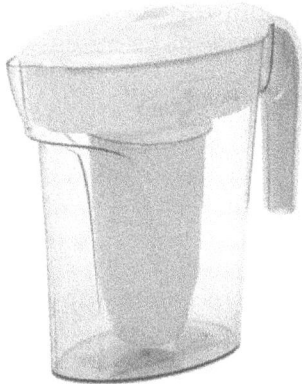

ZeroWater Pitcher-I
Tap water TDS is reduced from 100 ppm to 6 ppm.
This filter will last 3 to 4 weeks.

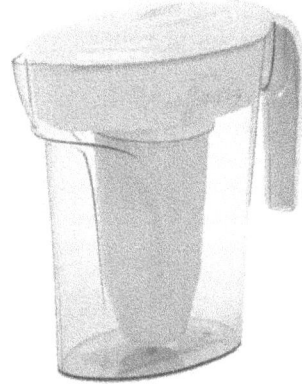

ZeroWater Pitcher-II
Filtered water TDS is reduced from 6 ppm to 0 ppm.
This filter will last a lot longer than 4 weeks.

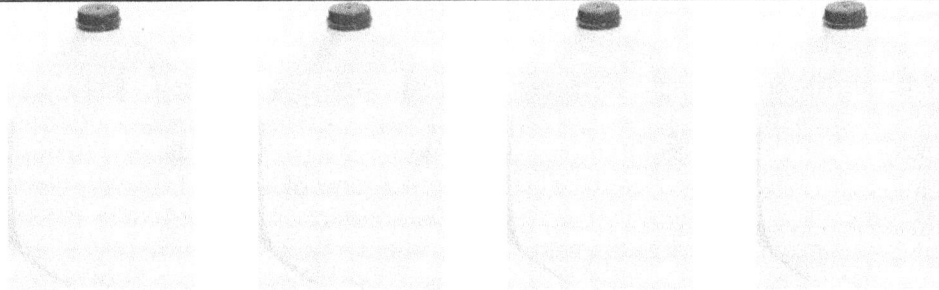

4-Liter Bottles Filled With Filtered Water (TDS = 6 ppm to 10 ppm, not drinkable)

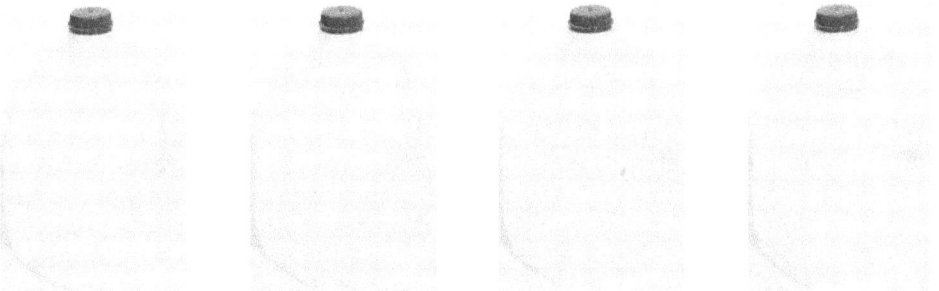

4-Liter Bottles Filled With Zero Water (TDS = 0 ppm, drinkable water)

Figure 14.4 How to use two ZeroWater filters simultaneously and save money.

WHY IS ZERO WATER PREFERABLE
COMPARED TO DISTILLED WATER AND RO WATER?

If it is manufactured, distributed and available in pristine condition, if it is genuine and trustworthy, and if it is one 100% free of contaminants, distilled water is the purest form of water (perfectly H2O), and is the best water for human consumption.

However under current day circumstances, the distilled water distribution industry is totally corrupt as it is very difficult to find the genuine distilled water in the market nowadays.

CHEAP HOME DISTILLERS ARE UNTRUSTWORTHY

◉ When you purchased a home distiller and started making your own distilled water, please get your distilled water tested by a local certified laboratory, and make sure that there are no contaminants present in the distilled water you made.

◉ CAUTION: Cheap home distillers can release contaminants from the materials of construction such as metal and/or plastic. Make sure that the home distiller's steam chamber, upper cover with condensing coil, fan and cap are properly designed and manufactured with the safe materials of construction so that the distilled water is free of contaminants.

◉ A customer purchased a home distiller on Amazon, and got his distilled water tested by a laboratory, and found elevated level of nickel contaminant. There was nothing he could do about it but stopped using that distiller. So please be careful when using home distillers.

STORE BOUGHT DISTILLED WATER IN BOTTLES IS UNTRUSTWORTHY

An innocent consumer can easily get into a trap by purchasing and drinking distilled water in bottles readily available all over the supermarkets. Bottled water is untrustworthy. Whenever you purchased distilled water or reverse osmosis water in bottles, make sure that it is genuinely purified water by testing it as explained below:

◉ **METHOD 1:** Dr. RK purchased and tested distilled water being sold in 4-liter bottles in Walmart, Real Canadian Superstore, Safeway and Save-On-Foods, in Vancouver area, British Columbia, Canada. He distilled this distilled water again in his home distiller. After the completion of the distillation process, there was a kind of colored, greasy and sticky SCUM deposited on the bottom of the distiller. It is dangerous to drink such distilled water. He had the same experience when he tested the reverse osmosis water (RO water).

◉ **METHOD 2:** He also boiled this distilled water in a stockpot with glass lid on the stove. He left the lid slightly opened so that the vapors would escape out. After all the distilled water is evaporated and escaped out, he found some golden brown colored scars (large scars and small scars) on the bottom of the stock pot. It is dangerous to drink such distilled water.

IF GENUINE DISTILLED WATER IS UNAVAILABLE, SWITCH TO ZERO WATER

◉ Distilled water is the purest form of water and is the best drinking water if it is available in its pristine condition. As explained above if the distilled water was tested and approved by a laboratory, you can drink it. If you are unable to purchase genuine distilled water or unable to make your own distilled water that is genuine, then please switch to zero water using a ZeroWater pitcher. ZeroWater filter removes 99.6% of dissolved solids from the tap water (everything is removed exactly as in distillation process).

TDS level of distilled water is 0 ppm. TDS level of zero water is also 0 ppm.

◉ When drinking zero water, learn how to remineralize and slightly alkalize zero water.

LEARN HOW TO REMINERALIZE AND SLIGHTLY ALKALIZE THE ZERO WATER

World Health Organization (WHO) reported that demineralized water (distilled water) leaches minerals from the body's cells, and develop many serious health risks including cancer and heart disease. This topic is discussed extensively in Appendix-13A (see below). Please refer to Chapter 17, Chapter 18 & Chapter 19 and learn how to remineralize and alkalize the purified water at home. There are experiments conducted at home.

RECOMMENDATIONS (by Dr. RK)

When you remineralize the zero water, please do not add too much Himalayan pink salt. Himalayan pink salt, Celtic sea salt or ConcenTrace mineral drops which contain extremely high quantity of sodium. Beware of that important information regarding the high sodium content. Research showed that many people who overconsumed sodium chloride (NaCl) beyond the RDA developed and suffered from hypertension, osteoporosis, kidney stones, Menierre's Syndrome (ear ringing), insomnia, motion sickness, asthma, and a variety of cancers. So learn how to add only a few kernels of Himalayan pink salt, Celtic sea salt so that the TDS level could be 50 ppm, 100 ppm, or maximum 200 ppm (Never exceed 200 ppm).

When you try to alkalize the zero water, please not add too much baking soda. If you do so, the pH will shoot up to 8.5. It is dangerous to drink water at pH=8.5 every day. Add only a few kernels of baking soda and measure pH. Let the pH be close to 7.

After making the zero water using ZeroWater pitcher, and after remineralizing and slightly alkalizing, boil the zero water using a glass kettle, store it in a glass bottle, and refrigerate it. Zero water because of its high purity should never be stored in metal containers. So make sure that you are not using any metal kettle.

When you boil the water, no matter what kind of water it is, pathogens (all kinds of bacteria, viruses, fungi, parasites), microorganisms and E. coli would be destroyed, and so you can drink the purified water worry-free.

Always drink zero water that is boiled and refrigerated, remineralized (up to a TDS level of 200 ppm, and slightly alkalized (pH=7 to 7.25).

RULE TO BE ADOPTED: Purfied water that is either neutralized (pH=7) or slightly alkalized (pH=7 to 7.25), and remineralized up to a TDS level of 200 ppm is the healthy drinking water.

Advantages of Zero Water Compared to Distilled Water

It takes 1 hour to make 1 liter of distilled water or 4 hour to make 4 liters of distilled water using a countertop home distiller, where as 1 liter of zero water can be made in 15 to 20 minutes using a Zerowater Pitcher or 4 liters of zero water can be made in 1 hour using a ZeroWater pitcher.

Countertop water distillers don't last long as they break down in a few weeks or few months where as ZeroWater Pitcher lasts long.

Zero water can be self-made at home. You can make your own zero water from tap water at the comfort of your home without depending on supermarkets or local delivery companies or other vendors. You don't have to purchase bottled water, which is untrustworthy.

DRAWBACKS OF ZEROWATER, BRITA & PUR FILTERS

These filters are not guaranteed to remove all contaminants from the tap water. They are designed to remove only some commonly found contaminants as listed on their websites.

You the consumer need to see your municipality's annual water quality report, and find out what contaminants are actually lurking in your tap water, and research and use an appropriate water purification system that is designed to remove the remaining contaminants (other than those removed by ZeroWater, Brita, or PUR filters).

BRITA WATER FILTRATION SYSTEM [5]

MAJOR DIFFERENCE BWTWEEN ZERO WATER FILTER & BRITA FILTER

While ZeroWater filter removes all contaminants from tap water and reduces the TDS level to zero, Brita® claims that their filters are meant to remove most commonly found contaminants (not all) from tap water, and that they are not committed to reduce the TDS level to zero.

Brita® claims that their products are tested and certified by the WQA (Water Quatoty Association) and also tested against NSF/ANSI Standards 42 and 53 for the reduction of the claims specified on the Performance Data Sheet. Brita® claims that their filters remove Lead, Mercury, Cadmium, Benzene, Asbestos, Particulates, Copper, Zinc, Tricholorobenzene, Select pharmaceuticals, pesticides/herbicides, TTHMs, Atrazine, and many other contaminants, making the tap water safe to drink. [5]

The major drawback of Brita® filter is that it is not certified to remove the dangerous contaminants (i) PFOA (perfluorooctanoic acid) and (ii) PFOS (perfluorooctane sulfonate).

Brita® manufactures and distributes a variety of pitchers, dispensers, faucet mounts: [5]

BRITA PITCHERS & DISPENSERS

(i) Brita® Colour Series Grand Pitcher
(ii) Brita® Marina Water Filtration Pitcher
(iii) Brita® Slim Water Filtration Pitcher

(iv) Brita® Soho Water Filtration Pitcher
(v) Brita® Space Saver Water Filtration Pitcher
(vi) Brita® Ultramax Dispenser with 1 Brita®

BRITA SINK FAUCET MOUNTS

(i) Brita® Faucet Mount Filtration Basic System - Chrome
(ii) Brita® Faucet Mount Filtration Basic System – White
In addition, Brita also sells "Carry-on Water Bottles" with filter inside.

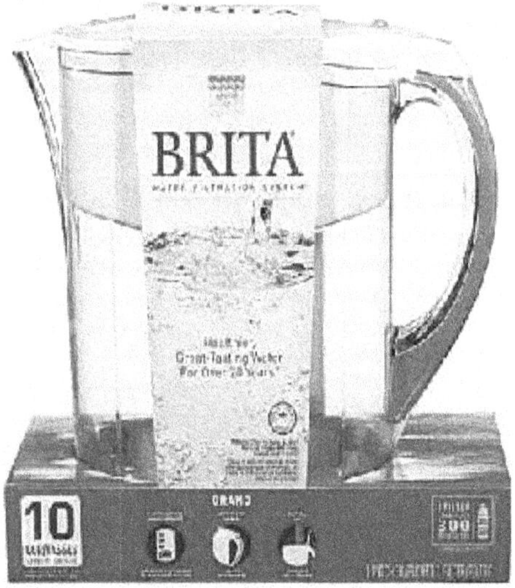

Courtesy of Brita®

Dr. RK personally tested the Brita Water Pitcher. He did the following experiment to test the Brita filtration unit. He purchased the Brita Water Pitcher in the local supermarket, and made purified water from tap water. He monitored the TDS level in the tap water and in the purified water obtained from Brita Water Pitcher. He noted the results of TDS carefully.

● For the tap water (in Burnaby, British Columbia, Canada), TDS = 22 ppm.
● For the purified water obtained from Brita Water Pitcher, TDS = 22 ppm.

CONCLUSION: Brita does not reduce TDS level in Canadian tap water. It might reduce TDS level in US tap water, if TDS level is very high, by 20%.

Figure 14.5 A typical Brita water filtration system to purify water.

PUR WATER FILTRATION SYSTEM [6]

Tap water may look clean, but can pick up potentially harmful contaminants and pollutants while traveling through very many zigzag pipelines before reaching your kitchen sink. So filtering your tap water before drinking is of utmost importance. PUR water pitcher filters are certified to reduce these chemical and physical contaminants, lurking in the tap water.

PUR pitcher filters and faucet filters are certified to reduce more contaminants than Brita's leading water filters, with easy tool-free installation. PUR's superior filtration technology removes 99 percent of lead and over 70 other contaminants, including 96% of Mercury and 92% of certain pesticides. Also reduces chlorine (taste and odour). Each PUR water filter gives you 30 gallons (480 Cups) of clean, healthy, great tasting water with unique Maxion filter technology by using activated carbon and ion exchange to reduce more contaminants than any other brand. The slim design of dispensers allows to fit comfortably in a fridge . [6]

PUR manufactures and distributes a variety of pitchers, dispensers, faucet mounts: [6]

PUR PITCHERS & DISPENSERS
(i) PUR 7-Cup Pitcher & (ii) PUrRPlus 7-Cup Pitcher
(iii) PUR 11-Cup Pitcher & (iv) PUR Plus 11-Cup Pitcher
(v) PUR 10-Cup Pitcher & (vi) PUR Plus 12-Cup Pitcher
(vii) PUR 18-Cup Dispenser & (viii) PUR 44-Cup Dispenser
(ix) PUR 30-Cup Dispenser & (x) PUR Plus 30-Cup Dispenser

PUR SINK FAUCET FILTERS
(i) PUR Faucet Filtration System, Vertical
(ii) PUR Faucet Filtration System, Horizontal
(iii) PUR Plus Faucet Filtration System, Horizontal
(iv) PUR Plus Faucet Filtration System, Horizontal with Bluetooth

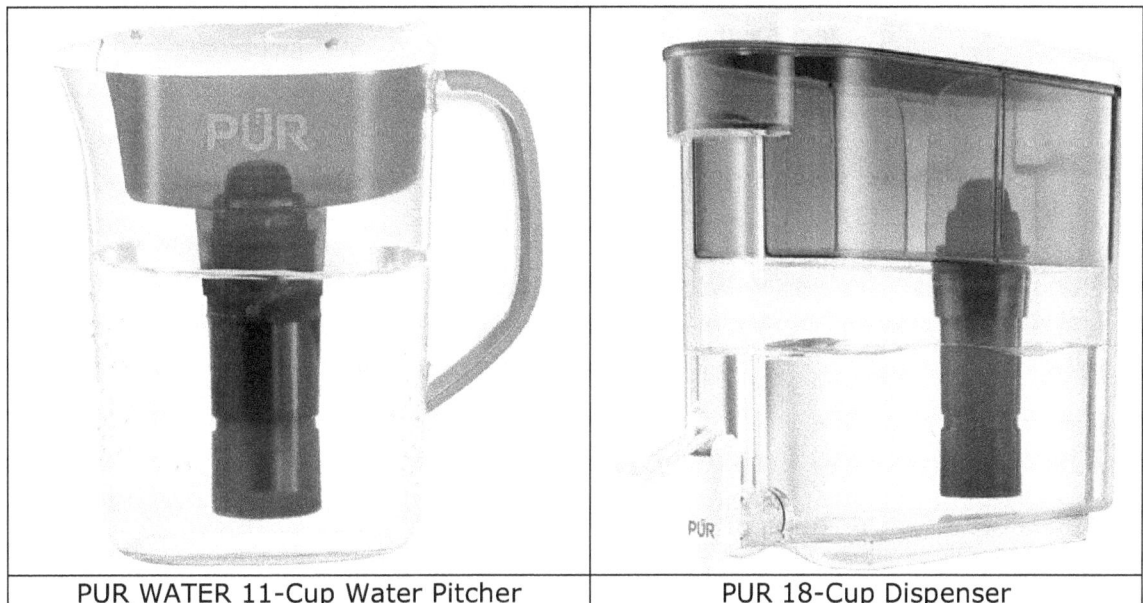

| PUR WATER 11-Cup Water Pitcher | PUR 18-Cup Dispenser |

Figure 14.6 PUR Water filtration systems to purify water (Courtesy of PUR).

AQUAGEAR WATER FILTRATION SYSTEM [7]

The Aquagear company claims that their filter with its robust filtering technology (proprietary blend of activated carbon and ion exchange media) catches contaminants like a magnet, and removes most dangerous impurities and toxins like PFOA/PFOS (Forever Chemicals), microplastics, lead, mercury, cadmium, copper, chlorine, asbestos, herbicides, pesticides, and trace pharmaceuticals, Volatile Organic Compounds (VOCs), and more.

Aquagear targets contaminants only without removing healthy minerals like calcium and magnesium. The Aquagear filter lasts up to 120 gallons of purified water. That is 3 times longer than competitor filters. Aquagear products are 100% BPA-free, lightweight, vegan, and recyclable.

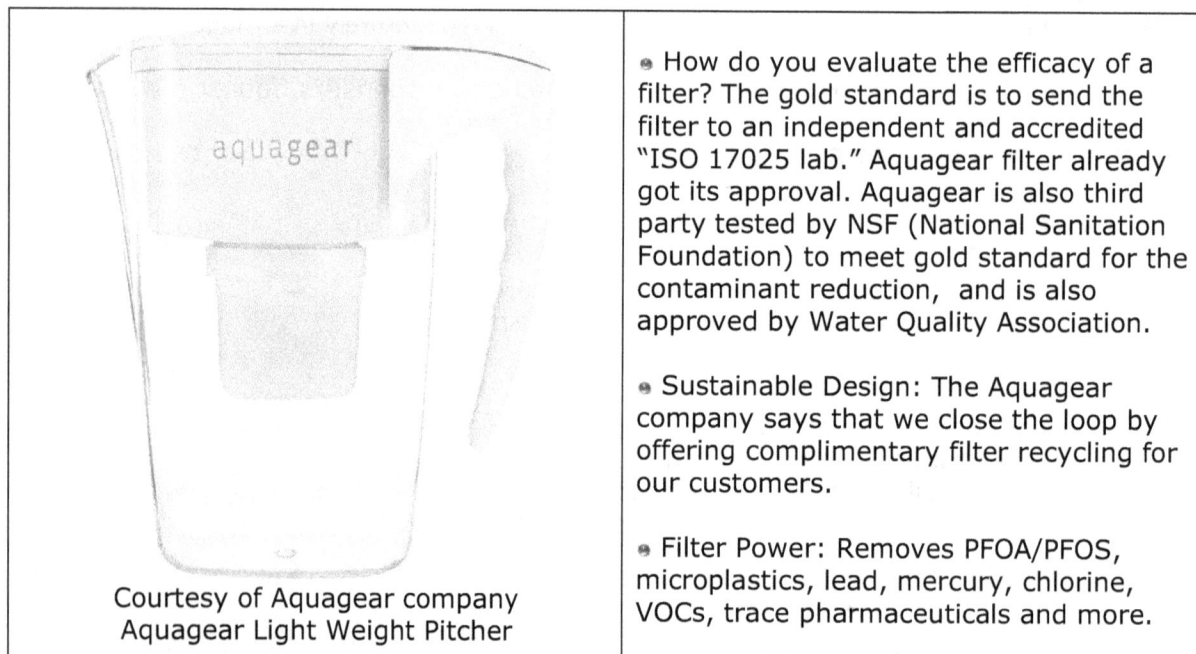

Courtesy of Aquagear company
Aquagear Light Weight Pitcher

● How do you evaluate the efficacy of a filter? The gold standard is to send the filter to an independent and accredited "ISO 17025 lab." Aquagear filter already got its approval. Aquagear is also third party tested by NSF (National Sanitation Foundation) to meet gold standard for the contaminant reduction, and is also approved by Water Quality Association.

● Sustainable Design: The Aquagear company says that we close the loop by offering complimentary filter recycling for our customers.

● Filter Power: Removes PFOA/PFOS, microplastics, lead, mercury, chlorine, VOCs, trace pharmaceuticals and more.

Figure 14.7 Aquagear Water filtration systems to purify water.

OTHER WATER FILTRATION SYSTEMS

(i) Nakii Water Filter, (ii) LARQ Water Bottles
(iii) Aquasana Water Filters, (iv) Waterdrop Under Sink Filters
(v) Kenmore Filters, (vi) Berkey Water Filters, (vii) Pure Aqua Water Filtration Systems
(viii) Culligan Reverse Osmosis Water Filters, (ix) Soma Water Filters
(x) Frigidaire Refrigerator Water Filtration System
and there are many other brands on tap water filtration.

● **IMPORTANT NOTE:** Do your own research thoroughly, and purchase and use a water filtration system that suits your purpose and interest. Request the "Water Quality Report" from the municipality of your local Government where you live, and by reading that report, learn how many contaminants could be present in the tap water, and find out a suitable filter that removes all or most of the contaminants. In addition, you should consider the fact that municipality water could pick up hidden contaminants while traveling through so many pipes before reaching your sink. In addition, you should consider the fact that plumbers could be working to repair pipes, and accidentally contaminated the water passing through pipelines. However it is important that you should never use tap water as the drinking water before you thoroughly purify it.

REFERENCES

1. ZeroWater Website.
https://zerowater.com/

2. PFAS (Perfluoroalkyl and Polyfluoroalkyl Substances) by NIH (National Institute of Environmental Health Sciences), Health and Education Section, Last Reviewed on November 17, 2021.
https://www.niehs.nih.gov/health/topics/agents/pfc/index.cfm

3. Performance Laboratiry Test Results (Compared to 2-Stage Filters).
https://zerowater.com/pages/results

4. ZeroWater Products (Pitchers to produce zero water at home).
https://zerowater.com/collections/all-water-filter-products

5. Brita Website
https://www.brita.com/
https://www.brita.com/why-brita/better-water/
https://www.brita.com/why-brita/better-water/

6. PUR website
https://www.pur.com/
https://www.pur.com/shop/pitchers
https://www.pur.com/shop/dispensers
https://www.pur.com/shop/faucet-systems

7. The Aquagear Filter
https://www.goaquagear.com/
https://www.goaquagear.com/pages/filter-performance

Bonus Reading from Chapter 17 & Chapter 18

**Remineralization and Alkalization Methods
Are Simplified and Explained Briefly in 2 Pages.**

By Reading These 2 Pages Only,
You Can Remineralize and Alkalize The Purified Water
(RO Water, Distilled Water, or Zero Water)
Like a Layperson at Home!

MAKE YOUR OWN NUTRITIOUS MINERAL WATER!
It Is Very Easy to Remineralize and Alkalize!
[You Don't Have to Read all Scientific Experiments!]

● However, you should adopt the following concept permanently into your mind: Purified water that is either neutralized (pH=7) or slightly alkalized (pH=7 to 7.25), and remineralized up to a TDS (Total Dissolved Solids) level of 200 ppm is the healthy drinking water!

HOW TO ALKALIZE AND REMINERALIZE LIKE A LAYPERSON

HOW TO SLIGHTLY ALKALIZE THE PURIFIED WATER LIKE A LAYPERSON

1. Fill up a glass bottle with 4 liters of purified water (RO water, distilled water, or zero water).
2. Add a tiny pinch of baking soda (only a few kernels), shake the bottle thoroughly, and measure the pH using one of the following items:
a. Enagic pH drops with color chart (you can purchase this at local Enagic store), or
b. pH test kit (pH drops) with color chart (you can purchase this in a pet store), or
c. Digital pH meter (practice and learn how to use this digital pH meter correctly).

⦿ If you add 3 drops of Enagic pH drops to a cup of slightly alkalized water, the water should turn green color. pH should be close to 7. If you add too much baking soda, pH shoots up to 8.5 (too alkaline). You should never drink such water with pH=8.5. You should always drink water with pH close to 7 (maximum 7.25).
⦿ By trial and error, and with practice, you will be able to add only a few kernels of baking soda, and will be able to adjust the purified water pH close to 7. It is very easy!
IMPORTANT NOTE: When you use baking soda to increase the pH of the purified water, you must do urine test frequently and make sure that your urine pH is under 8.

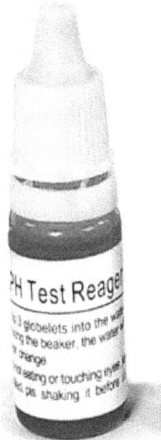

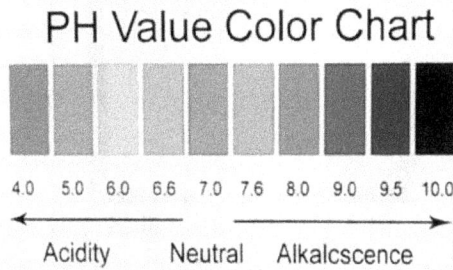

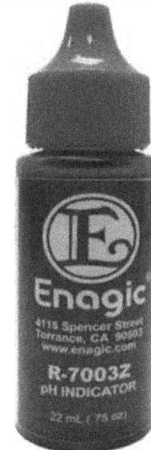

PH Value Color Chart

| 4.0 | 5.0 | 6.0 | 6.6 | 7.0 | 7.6 | 8.0 | 9.0 | 9.5 | 10.0 |

Acidity   Neutral   Alkalescence

a. On the right is the Enagic pH Testing Drops.   Courtesy of Enagic Co.
b. On the Left is pH Testing Reagent Drops with color chart to measure the water pH.

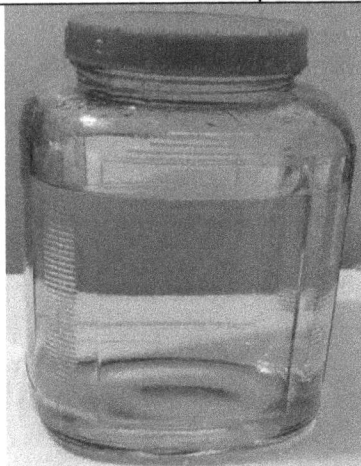

Glass Bottle Filled With 4 Liters of Purified Water.

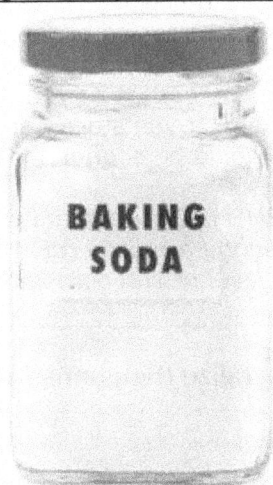

Baking Soda

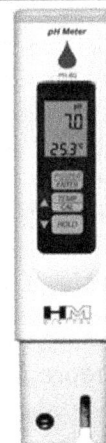

c. Digital pH meter Courtesy of H.M. Digital.

Figure 17.1 How to alkalize the purified water like a layperson.

HOW TO REMINERALIZE THE PURIFIED WATER LIKE A LAYPERSON
[Continued from Previous page]

1. You have just alkalized the purified water (RO water, distilled water, or zero water) by adding a tiny pinch of baking soda so that pH is close to 7, as explained in previous page .
2. You now remineralize this same water by adding a tiny pinch (only a few kernels) of Himalayan pink salt or Celtic sea salt into the same glass bottle of purified water without using digital kitchen scale, but with your fingers. After adding salt, shake the bottle thoroughly in a circular motion so that all the purified water is remineralized.
3. Monitor the TDS level using a TDS meter. Make sure that the TDS level is 20 ppm, 50 ppm, 100 ppm, or 150 ppm (your desired TDS level). Some people like 20 ppm, and some others like 50 ppm or 100 ppm. Add more Himalayan pink salt (only a few kernels) if the TDS level is below your desired level. Do not exceed TDS=200 ppm.

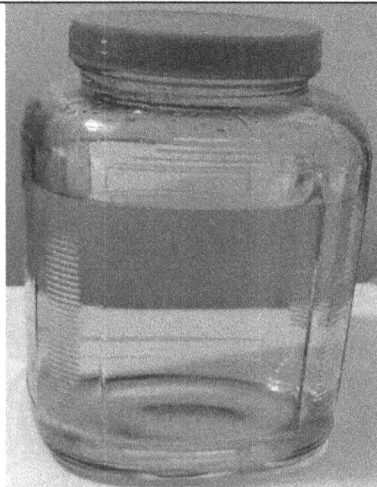

Glass Bottle Filled With 4-Liters of Purified Water.

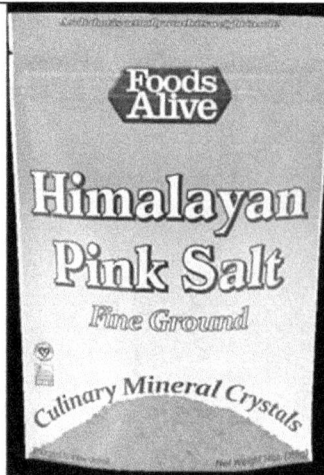

Himalayan pink salt, Or Celtic Sea salt

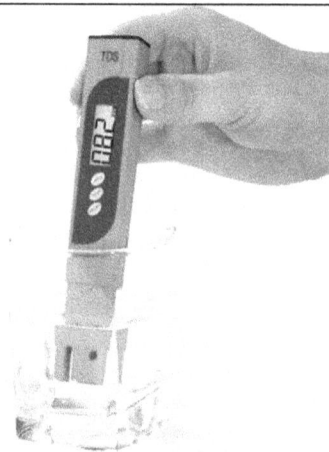

TDS Meter
Courtesy of H. M. Digital

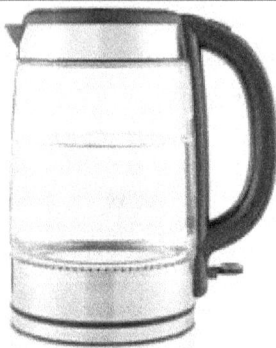

4. Boil this purified water that is remineralized and slightly alkalized using a glass kettle (do not use metal kettle).
5. Store this boiled water in 4-liter glass bottles, and leave them to be cooled to room temperature.
6. Then transfer this cold water into a 4-liter plastic bottles (as many bottles as you wish), and refrigerate it before drinking. If you store water in FOUR 4-liter plastic bottles, that would be enough for a week (if you drink 8 cups a day).

● *REMEMBER: Purified water that is either neutralized (pH=7) or slightly alkalized (pH= 7 to 7.5), and remineralized up to a TDS level of 200 ppm is the healthy drinking water.*

Glass Kettle (1.7 Liters)

Figure 17.2 How to remineralize the purified water like a layperson.

You Have Just Learned How to Remineralize and Alkalize the Purified Water Like A Layperson Without Measuring the Salt Content Precisely Using A Digital Kitchen Scale!

If You Want to Read About the Scientific Experiments Conducted Using A Digital Kitchen Scale, TDS Meter and Digital pH Meter, Please Purchase and Read the Book (i) Drinking Water Guide, or (ii) Drinking Water Guide-II

CHAPTER 17	REMINERALIZATION OF THE PURIFIED WATER ▷ How to Remineralize the Purified Water at Home?
CHAPTER 18	ALKALINE WATER ▷ How to Alkalize the Purified Water at Home?
CHAPTER 19	DRINKING WATER GUIDE IN A NETSHELL ▷ QUICK-REFERENCE & DOI-IT-YOURSELF GUIDELINES

THE PURPOSE OF THE BOOK "THE ORIGIN OF THE EARTH'S WATER" FULFILLED

⏺ OUR UNIVERSE, OUR STARS, OUR MILKY WAY GALAXY, OUR SOLAR SYSTEM, OUR SUN, OUR PLANET EARTH, OUR MOON & OUR WATER: How Were They Created? This book has answered that question in a simple layperson's language.

⏺ The purpose of Chapter 1 & Chapter 20 is to let everybody know where exactly our planet Earth is located in our Universe, and how exactly our planet Earth possessed that much liquid water that we drink to survive today. This objective has been fulfilled through an extensive research, innovative depictions, mindful clarification, and the scientific evidence gathered by astronomers, cosmologists, space scientists and researchers. The Origin of the Earth's Water revealed briefly in Chapter 1!

⏺ In Chapter 20, "The Origin of the Earth's Water" expanded with all the research details including scientific journal publications. Astronomers, space researchers, scientists and very many academic researchers have been struggling to find out the truth through out the human history, but were unable to come up with a definitive answer thus far. However all those scientific research findings are summarized in Chapter 20, and clarified that our Earth inherited up to 50% of its water from the interstellar medium, and obtained the rest of the water from the bombardment of Asteroids. The book provided the proof how researchers eliminated "Comets" as the source of water formation.

⏺ **This book unveiled the truth about water formation on our planet Earth:** Water [H_2O] is made from two hydrogen atoms and one oxygen atom. Water forms anywhere in our Milky Way Galaxy and in our Universe as long as the appropriate conditions prevail:
(i) Both hydrogen and oxygen must abundantly be available under appropriate climate conditions (temperature below -223 °C or 50 °K is necessary in most cases), and
(ii) the ionization of hydrogen molecules should readily be possible in order to take place the chemical reaction.
The primary element hydrogen was first created nearly 380,000 years after the Big Bang when our Universe was just born. But oxygen was not available in our Universe until and after some 400 million years when the first stars were born. After the stars formation commenced, both hydrogen and oxygen were abundantly available throughout our Universe and more specifically in our Milky Way Galaxy. Oxygen is made in stars when the primitive elements such as hydrogen, helium and lithium were fused to form many other heavier elements, and dispersed out into our Universe in events such as supernova explosions. The two elements "hydrogen and oxygen" react in star-forming clouds and form large amounts of water [$2 H_2 + O_2 = 2 H_2O$]. The molecules of water leave the clouds of dust and gas, and end up in many different places – planets, comets, asteroids, and meteorites. And that is how our Earth inherited water even before it was born. Our Earth was thus born with water.

⏺ In Chapter 14, this book also teaches how to alkalize and remineralize the zero water at home. Just by reading the instructions provided in 2 pages only, you will be able to remineralize and alkalize the purified water (RO water, distilled water, or zero water) like a layperson.

LIVE LIKE AN ADVANCED HUMAN BEING!
⏺ Please do not drink tap water, well water, or bottled water of any kind directly without knowing how pure it is. Please always drink purified water (reverse osmosis water, distilled water, or zero water), and learn how to neutralize it or slightly alkalize it, and remineralize it before drinking.
⏺ Purified water that is either neutralized (pH=7) or slightly alkalized (pH=7 to 7.25), and remineralized up to a TDS (Total Dissolved Solids) level of 200 ppm is the healthy drinking water.

⏺ REMEMBER: More than 99% of your amazing body's molecules are water molecules, and 55% to 60% of your body weight is water. You therefore should make sure that the water in your body is clean, healthy and nutritious, and more importantly you should make sure that the water you drink is one hundred percent free of contaminants! This book is designed to help you achieve that goal!

About the Author

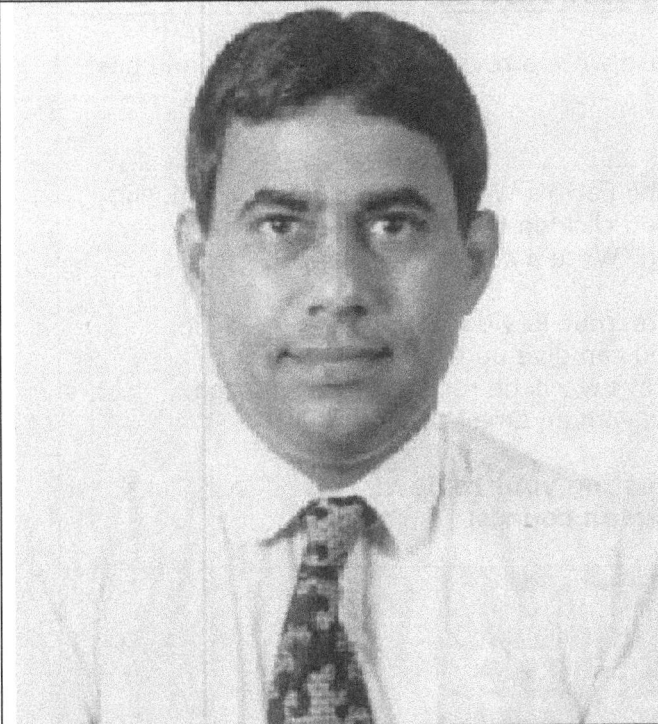

Dr. Rao M Konduru was a Chemical Engineer, and held two Master's degrees and two doctorates and two post-doctoral titles, all in chemical engineering. He published a book in 2003 titled "Permanent Diabetes Control," which earned immense respect and appreciation. Many people said it was a wonderful book. After suffering from a sudden heart attack in 1998, even though his left artery was 75% clogged with severe angina, he said "NO" to bypass surgery. He did what none of us would even think of doing. He simply relied on his natural self-prevention diet and exercise, and with it he reversed his critical diabetic heart disease in a matter of months, and developed a method to accomplish Permanent Diabetes Control. He also came up with a trial-and-error procedure to determine the optimal insulin dose that would tightly control diabetes, and would allow a diabetic person to live like a normal person for the rest of his/her life.

Dr. Rao M Konduru maintained his hemoglobin A1c level under 6.0% consistently. His personal best hemoglobin A1c level of 5.0% was an extraordinary result any diabetic person would hope to accomplish in a lifetime. Perhaps Dr. Rao M Konduru was the only diabetic person lived in this world with "Permanent Diabetes Control".

Once again, health demons such as uncontrollable weight gain, sleep apnea and chronic insomnia came his way. He did not give up, but persisted on discovering new, natural and effortless treatments of his own in reversing these most difficult disorders. His extensive scientific research experience and his powerful knowledge helped him battle and combat these life challenges. He figured out their root causes, and developed natural yet powerful techniques to cure these health disorders himself. After losing 40 pounds of weight and 12 inches around the waist, he successfully reversed his obesity, obstructive sleep apnea and chronic insomnia. He carefully created and published the following excellent guidebooks on Amazon so that others can benefit and be inspired to achieve similar results. His most recent book "Drinking Water Guide" is a 540-page book of wealth of information on drinking water for the rest of us.

1. Permanent Diabetes Control	www.mydiabetescontrol.com
2. The Secret to Controlling Type 2 Diabetes	www.mydiabetescontrol.com
3. Reversing Obesity	www.reversingsleepapnea.com/ebook2.html
4. Reversing Sleep Apnea	www.reversingsleepapnea.com
5. Reversing Insomnia	www.reversinginsomnia.com
6. Reversing Insomnia in 3 Days	www.reversinginsomnia.com
7. Drinking Water Guide	www.drinkingwaterguide.com
8. Drinking Water Guide-II	www.drinkingwaterguide.com
9. The Origin of the Earth's Water	www.drinkingwaterguide.com
10. Autobiography Of Dr. Rao M Konduru	www.mydiabetescontrol.com/Bio/

- Prime Publishing Co.

PLEASE WRITE A REVIEW ABOUT THIS BOOK

Now that you have read this book, please write a review about this book, and post your review on Amazon.

a. Please log into your Amazon account,
b. Search for this book "The Origin of the Earth's Water (Author: Rao Konduru, PhD)", or by using ISBN # 9780973112085, and click on the book cover & scroll down,
c. Click on "Customer Reviews", click on "Write a customer review" button, and "Create Review" box pops up.
d. Kindly write your REVIEW in the Write-Your-Review box, type a Headline, and click on 5 stars overall rating (you can give up to 5 stars).
e. Click on "Submit" button, and your review will be registered on Amazon.
f. Amazon will acknowledge your review with an email confirmation!

Thanks for posting your review!
Your opinion counts!

YOUR OPINION COUNTS!

Kindle eBook Is Available on Amazon

You can read this book on your computer, laptop, tablet, e-reader, iPhone, or any Kindle device by purchasing Kindle eBook. It is available on Amazon. Please log into your Amazon account, and search for "The Origin of the Earth's Water, Kindle eBook", or ASIN # B0844LWRB1

THE END OF THE BOOK "THE ORIGIN OF THE EARTH'S WATER"!

BEST WISHES!

www.ingramcontent.com/pod-product-compliance
Lightning Source LLC
Chambersburg PA
CBHW081415270326
41931CB00015B/3289